# The EKG Handbook

**THERESA ANN MIDDLETON BROSCHE, MSN, BSN, RN, CCRN**

**JEFFREY L. WILLIAMS, MD, MS, FACC**
*Reviewer*
Director
The Good Samaritan Health System
Lebanon Cardiology Associates, PC
Lebanon County, Pennsylvania

**JONES AND BARTLETT PUBLISHERS**
*Sudbury, Massachusetts*
BOSTON     TORONTO     LONDON     SINGAPORE

D1262775

*World Headquarters*
Jones and Bartlett Publishers
40 Tall Pine Drive
Sudbury, MA 01776
978-443-5000
info@jbpub.com
www.jbpub.com

Jones and Bartlett Publishers
Canada
6339 Ormindale Way
Mississauga, Ontario L5V 1J2
Canada

Jones and Bartlett Publishers
International
Barb House, Barb Mews
London W6 7PA
United Kingdom

Jones and Bartlett's books and products are available through most bookstores and online booksellers. To contact Jones and Bartlett Publishers directly, call 800-832-0034, fax 978-443-8000, or visit our website, www.jbpub.com.

Substantial discounts on bulk quantities of Jones and Bartlett's publications are available to corporations, professional associations, and other qualified organizations. For details and specific discount information, contact the special sales department at Jones and Bartlett via the above contact information or send an email to specialsales@jbpub.com.

The authors, editor, and publisher have made every effort to provide accurate information. However, they are not responsible for errors, omissions, or for any outcomes related to the use of the contents of this book and take no responsibility for the use of the products and procedures described. Treatments and side effects described in this book may not be applicable to all people; likewise, some people may require a dose or experience a side effect that is not described herein. Drugs and medical devices are discussed that may have limited availability controlled by the Food and Drug Administration (FDA) for use only in a research study or clinical trial. Research, clinical practice, and government regulations often change the accepted standard in this field. When consideration is being given to use of any drug in the clinical setting, the health care provider or reader is responsible for determining FDA status of the drug, reading the package insert, and reviewing prescribing information for the most up-to-date recommendations on dose, precautions, and contraindications, and determining the appropriate usage for the product. This is especially important in the case of drugs that are new or seldom used.

**Production Credits**
Publisher: Kevin Sullivan
Aquisitions Editor: Emily Ekle
Aquisitions Editor: Amy Sibley
Associate Editor: Patricia Donnelly
Editorial Assistant: Rachel Shuster
Associate Production Editor: Amanda Clerkin
Marketing Manager: Rebecca Wasley
V.P., Manufacturing and Inventory Control: Therese Connell
Composition: Paw Print Media
Cover Design: Scott Moden
Printing and Binding: Malloy, Inc.
Cover Printing: Malloy, Inc.

6048

Printed in the United States of America
13 12 11 10 09   10 9 8 7 6 5 4 3 2 1

**Library of Congress Cataloging-in-Publication Data**
Brosche, Theresa.
  The EKG handbook / Theresa Brosche.
    p. ; cm.
  Includes bibliographical references and index.
  ISBN-13: 978-0-7637-6995-6 (alk. paper)
  ISBN-10: 0-7637-6995-9 (alk. paper)
  1. Electrocardiography—Handbooks, manuals, etc. I. Title.
  [DNLM: 1. Electrocardiography—methods—Handbooks. 2. Electrocardiography—methods—Nurses' Instruction. 3. Heart Diseases—diagnosis—Handbooks. 4. Heart Diseases—diagnosis—Nurses' Instruction. WG 39 B874e 2010]
  RC683.5.E5B726 2010
  616.1'207547—dc22
                    2009012323

# Acknowledgments

I would like to begin by thanking Jeffrey Williams, MD, MS, FACC from Lebanon Cardiology Associates for taking the time to review the book and providing an expert analysis of the material.

I would like to thank my husband and my children, Scott, Ben, and Matthew, for their support and their patience, and my parents, Susie and Charlie, for their encouragement and inspiration. In particular, I would like to thank my mother, a cardiac nurse for the past 40-plus years, who has shared her passion for electrocardiography with me and to whom I owe so much.

I would also like to acknowledge and thank David Morris, BS, NRENT-P, Emily Ekle, and all of the editorial staff of Jones and Bartlett for their enthusiastic and positive support, direction, and editorial assistance.

Finally, and most importantly, I would like to thank God for His many blessings and for being by my side throughout the writing and production phases of this handbook.

—Theresa Ann Middleton Brosche

# Contents

# Preface

*"Passion for electrocardiography can only increase as one gains a greater understanding of the unique electrical conduction patterns of the heart."*

This handbook is designed to provide practical, up-to-date information for the novice, the advanced student, or the clinician to assist in identifying and analyzing rhythm strips as well as exploring other major topics related to the EKG.

The book is presented in two parts:

- The first part of the handbook presents the basic components of the EKG:
  - Action potential
  - Depolarization
  - Repolarization
  - Normal and abnormal electrical activity of the heart
  - EKG monitoring systems
  - Tips to obtain the "best picture"
  - Measuring, calculating, and documenting
  - A six-step method for analyzing the 12-lead EKG
  - An eight-step method for analyzing rhythm strips

- The second part of the handbook presents the rhythms:
  - 30-plus rhythms
  - Tips to assist in differentiating certain rhythms from one another
  - Figures, definitions, and a practical application of the eight-step method are used in this section to assist the reader in understanding, analyzing, and evaluating the rhythms

The layout of the book was inspired by my students, who continually look for ways to connect the dots between what they read and what they see. Although the book is by no means all-inclusive of the plethora of information related to EKGs, my goal is to provide the reader with essential information that will lead to a greater understanding of the unique electrical conduction patterns of the heart and will assist in the interpretation of EKGs.

The information is presented in a concise, compact, easy-to-read format using figures, tables, and bullets. The handbook can fit easily into lab coats, jackets, school desks, and book bags for use while at work, at home, or at school.

I hope you enjoy this book as much as I have enjoyed writing it. Thank you for the opportunity to share my passion for electrocardiography with you.

Yours Truly,

*Theresa Ann Middleton Brosche*

Theresa Ann Middleton Brosche
*Adjunct Clinical Faculty*
*Germanna Community College*
*Spotsylvania, Virginia*
*Mary Washington Hospital*
*Fredericksburg, Virginia*

# Foreword

*The EKG Handbook*, by Terry Brosche, MSN, BSN, RN, CCRN, is a great addition to the body of work on electrocardiography. From basic concepts about the cardiac action potential to AV node reentrant tachycardia, her book balances simplicity with complexity in an attempt to distill this field (that many spend decades mastering) into a manageable introductory monograph. Better yet, the author manages to provide a completely referenced text so that readers can dig deeper into electrocardiography whether they are interested in the origin of U waves or how to calculate QT intervals in patients with atrial fibrillation. As we move forward over the next several decades and cardiac disease explodes in prevalence, it is more important than ever to offer our healthcare students the most comprehensive and widely varied electrocardiography texts that are suited to their learning styles.

Jeffrey L. Williams, MD, MS, FACC
*Director, Clinical Cardiac Electrophysiology*
*The Good Samaritan Health System*
*Lebanon Cardiology Associates, PC*

# SECTION 1

# Brief Review of the Anatomy of the Heart

- The adult heart weighs approximately 0.75 lb and is protected by the sternum, the spinal column, and the lungs (Gersh, 2000).
- The heart is surrounded by the pericardium. The outer layer is called the parietal pericardium, and the inner layer is called the visceral pericardium. In between these layers is a small amount of serous fluid that acts as a lubricant and allows the two membranes to slide easily over one another with each heartbeat (Clark, 2005).
- The heart wall is composed of three layers:
  - Epicardium: The outer layer of the heart wall.
  - Myocardium: The middle and largest portion of the heart wall.
  - Endocardium: The innermost layer of the heart wall (see Figure 1-1).
- The heart is located to the left of the center of the chest and is shaped like a cone with the lower part of the heart, called the apex, resting on the upper surface of the diaphragm (Stewart & Vitello-Cicciu, 1996).
- The upper part of the heart, called the base, tilts slightly backwards toward the spinal column, and from it emerges the pulmonary trunk and the aorta.
- The anatomical position of the right side of the heart is toward the front of the chest.
- The anatomical position of the left side of the heart is toward the back of the chest.

> *Note:* The muscular wall of the left ventricle is larger than the muscular wall of the right ventricle. This is because the pressure in the systemic circulation, which the left ventricle pumps against, is much higher than the pressure in the pulmonic circulation, which the right ventricle pumps against (Smith, 1996).

**Figure 1-1 The pericardium and the three layers of the heart**

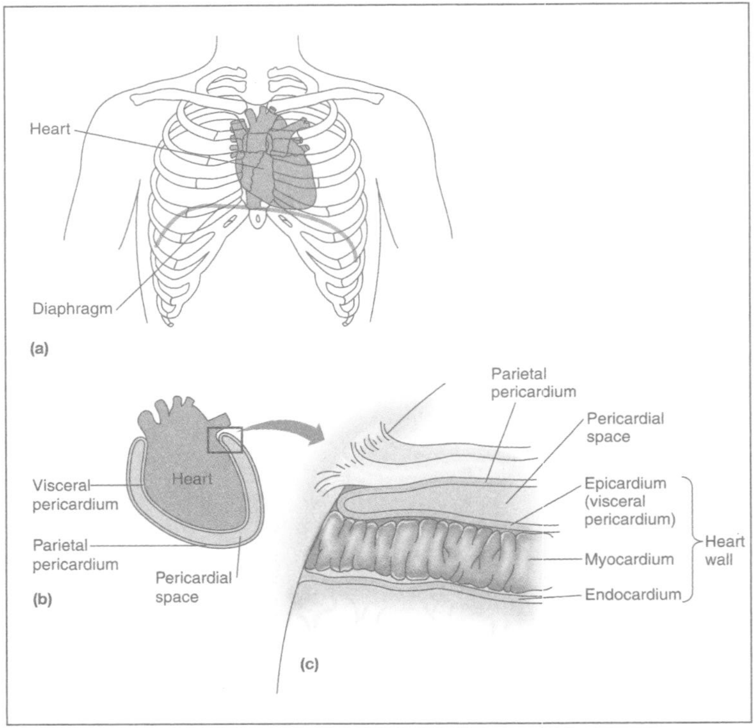

Source: Clark, R. K. *Human Anatomy Flash Cards: Skeletal and Muscular Systems.* © 2005 by Jones and Bartlett Publishers.

- A septum separates the right side of the heart from the left side of the heart.
- The heart has four chambers and four valves that work in harmony to keep the blood flowing in one direction from the right side of the heart to the left side of the heart.
  - The four chambers of the heart are:
    - Right atrium
    - Right ventricle
    - Left atrium
    - Left ventricle
  - The four valves of the heart consist of:
    - Two atrioventricular (AV) valves that allow the blood to flow between the chambers of the heart. (Papillary muscles attached to the chordae tendineae of the AV valves keep the valves closed during ventricular contraction.)
      - ✓ Tricuspid valve: The tricuspid valve sits between the right atrium and the right ventricle.
      - ✓ Mitral valve: The mitral valve sits between the left atrium and the left ventricle. (The mitral valve is also called the bicuspid valve.)
    - Two semilunar valves that allow the blood to flow out of the heart.
      - ✓ Pulmonic valve: The pulmonic valve connects the right ventricle to the pulmonic circulation.
      - ✓ Aortic valve: The aortic valve connects the left ventricle to the systemic circulation.

> *Note:* The valves of the heart open and close because of pressure changes within the chambers of the heart. For example, the tricuspid and the mitral valves will snap shut (at the same time) when the pressure in the ventricles exceeds the pressure in the atria. The aortic and pulmonic valves will snap shut (at the same time) when the arterial pressure within the pulmonic trunk and the aorta exceeds the pressure within the ventricle. The closure of the valves is what produces the heart sounds lub dub.

## BLOOD FLOW THROUGH THE HEART

Please refer to Figures 1-2 and 1-3 for diagrams of the blood flow through the heart.

- Deoxygenated blood from the systemic circulation enters the right atrium and then travels through the tricuspid valve to the right ventricle.
- This deoxygenated blood is pumped from the right ventricle through the pulmonic valve, into the left and right pulmonary arteries, and then into the lungs.
- While in the lungs, the blood becomes oxygenated and then travels through the pulmonary veins to the left atrium.
- Oxygenated blood from the left atrium travels through the mitral valve to the left ventricle, then through the aortic valve, and into the aorta, where it travels to the systemic circulation.
- This blood flow is affected by the electrical conduction system of the heart, which provides the "electrical energy" so the heart can pump the blood.

## CARDIAC OUTPUT

- Cardiac output is the amount of blood ejected by the heart into the systemic circulation each minute. To calculate the cardiac output, multiply the heart rate times the stroke volume.

> *Note:* Stroke volume is the amount of blood ejected by the heart into the systemic circulation with each ventricular contraction.

- The normal cardiac output is 4–8 l/min (Diepenbrock, 2004).
- If the heart rate or the stroke volume is reduced, the patient's cardiac output will be reduced.
- A reduction in cardiac output can negatively impact blood flow to the systemic circulation.

**Figure 1-2    Technical look at the structure and blood flow through the heart**

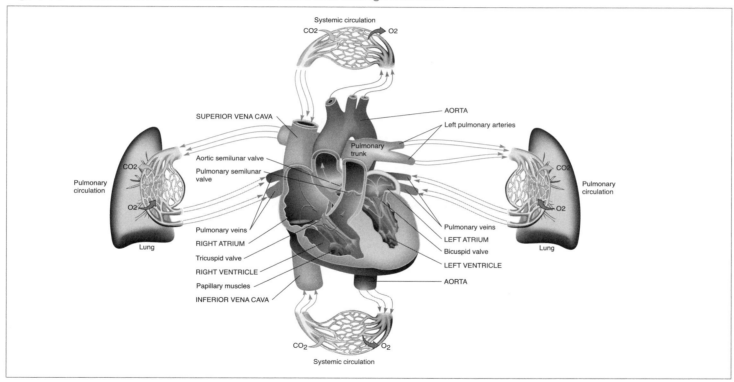

*Source*: Jackson, J. & Jackson, L. *Clinical nursing pocket guide*. Jones and Bartlett Publishers.

**Figure 1-3    Simplistic look at the structure and blood flow through the heart**

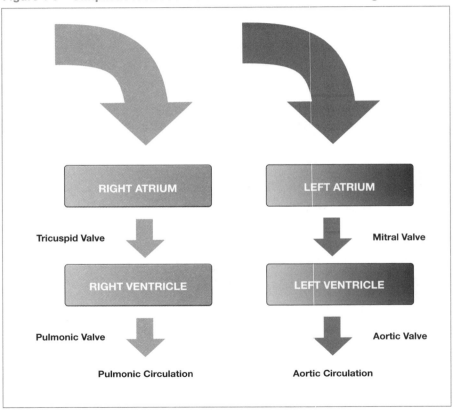

# SECTION 2

# Depolarization

- In normal physiology the muscle of the heart, also known as the myocardium, depolarizes when an exchange of electrically charged ions alters the electronegative gradient that exists within the myocardial cell (Twedell, 2005).
- Depolarization is represented by a QRS complex on the electrocardiogram (ECG).

**Figure 2-1    Depolarization and a QRS complex**

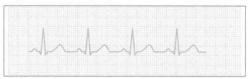

*Source*: Jackson, J. & Jackson, L. *Clinical nursing pocket guide*. Jones and Bartlett Publishers.

# SECTION 3

# Repolarization

- In normal physiology the myocardium recovers or repolarizes when the exchange of electrically charged ions restores the electronegative gradient back to the resting or restorative state within the myocardial cell.
- The heart spends a greater amount of time repolarizing than depolarizing.
- Repolarization is represented by a T wave on the EKG.

## REPOLARIZATION AND THE ABSOLUTE AND RELATIVE REFRACTORY TIME

Please refer to Figure 3-1 for absolute and relative refractory time.

- During repolarization there is a period of time when the heart cannot react to an electrical impulse. This is called the absolute refractory period.
- There is also a period of time during the latter part of repolarization when the heart may be responsive to an electrical impulse. This is called the relative refractory period.
- It is during the relative refractory period that the heart is most vulnerable because an electrical stimulus can fire into the T wave causing a lethal ventricular arrhythmia.

**Figure 3-1   Absolute and relative refractory time**

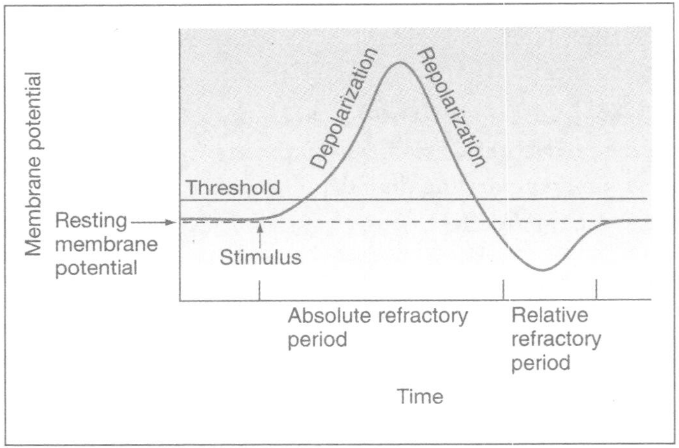

Source: Clark, R. K. *Human Anatomy Flash Cards: Skeletal and Muscular Systems.* © 2005 by Jones and Bartlett Publishers.

# Action Potential of the Cardiac Cell, Depolarization, and Repolarization

- The action potential is created by an exchange of electrically charged ions across the cardiac cell membrane.
- The exchange of ions during each phase of the action potential alters the electrical potential or internal charge of the cell, causing either depolarization or repolarization.
- The action potential in the nonpacemaker cardiac cell has five phases beginning with phase 0 and ending with phase 4 (see Figures 4-1 and 4-2).

**Sodium and Potassium**

Sodium is the primary extracellular ion, and potassium is the primary intracellular ion. An imbalance in the levels of these ions can alter the electrical potential of the cell and can increase the patient's susceptibility to arrhythmias.

**Figure 4-1   Shift in sodium and potassium ions during the action potential of the cell**

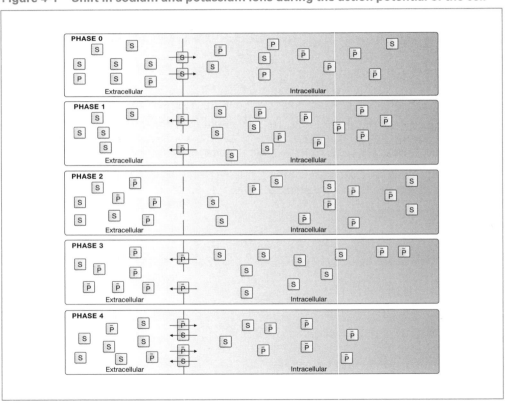

**Figure 4-2   Phases of the action potential**

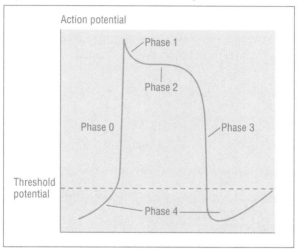

*Source*: From *12-Lead ECG: The Art of Interpretation*, courtesy of Tomas B. Garcia, MD.

**Box 4-1    Five phases of Action Potential in the Nonpacemaker Cardiac Cells**

✓ Phase Zero: Depolarization.
  • Sodium rushes into the cell and changes the internal charge of the cell from negative to positive.
  • Antiarrhythmic drugs that affect Phase 0 by slowing depolarization include:
    – Quinidine
    – Procainamide
    – Disopyramide
    – Lidocaine
    – Flecanide
    – Propafenone
✓ Phase One: Early repolarization.
  • Sodium channels partially close, potassium begins to leave the cell, and the internal charge of the cell becomes negative.
✓ Phase Two: Plateau phase.
  • Although potassium continues to move out of the cell, there is very little exchange of ions during this time and the internal charge remains relatively constant (Langfitt, 1984, p. 107).
✓ Phase Three: Final and rapid phase of repolarization.
  • The greatest amount of potassium is lost from the cell during this phase and the sodium channels are inactivated. The internal charge of the cell becomes more negative.
  • Amiodarone and Phase three:
    – Amiodarone blocks the sodium, potassium, and calcium channels causing a delay in repolarization of the cell and a prolonged action potential (Win-Kuang, 2000).
✓ Phase Four: Resting or restorative phase.
  • Sodium and potassium are exchanging positions across the cell membrane with the help of the sodium-potassium pump.
  • The sodium-potassium pump transports excess sodium from the inside of the cell to the outside of the cell. It also moves potassium from the outside of the cell back to the inside of the cell. By restoring ionic concentrations inside and outside of the cell, the electronegative gradient is reestablished and the process can begin again.

**Figure 4-3   Ventricular Fibrillation**

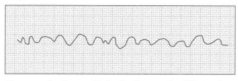

*Source*: Jackson, J. & Jackson, L. *Clinical nursing pocket guide*. Jones and Bartlett Publishers.

## DANGER ZONE

- The interval from the midpoint of phase 3 to just prior to phase 4 is called the relative refractory period, and it corresponds to the period in which the greatest amount of potassium is lost from the cell.
- During this period of time, the repolarizing heart can be stimulated inappropriately by an electrical stimulus, which can lead to a lethal ventricular arrhythmia called ventricular fibrillation (see Figure 4-3).

## ACTION POTENTIAL OF THE PACEMAKER CELLS OF THE HEART

The action potential of the pacemaker cells of the heart (sinus node, AV node, and the Purkinje network) differs from the action potential of the nonpacemaker cells of the heart (nonpacemaker cells are all the other myocardial cells throughout the heart) in the following ways:

- The calcium ion plays an important role in altering the electrical charge within the pacemaker cell.
- The electrical charge within the pacemaker cell never becomes positive; it becomes more or less negative. This is what enables the pacemaker cells to be more likely to initiate an action potential and to depolarize spontaneously.

# SECTION 5

# Myocardial Cells or Myocytes

- Each myocardial cell within the heart has the ability to initiate an electrical impulse, to respond to an electrical impulse, to transmit an electrical impulse, and to cause pumping action within the heart muscle. These actions are referred to as:
  - Automaticity-initiate
  - Excitability-respond
  - Conductivity-transmit
  - Contractility-pumping action

## ABNORMAL CONDITION OF THE MYOCARDIAL CELLS: ECTOPIC BEAT

- An ectopic beat is a beat that originates from an abnormal focus, i.e., a focus other than the sinoatrial (SA) node. (Refer to Section 6).
- This abnormal focus can occur anywhere within the heart if not suppressed by the natural pacemaker cells of the heart.
- An ectopic beat can originate from one site or from multiple sites within the heart, producing a single isolated beat, grouped beats, or an arrhythmia (Pugh, 2000, p. 565; see Figure 5-1).

## CAUSES OF ECTOPIC BEATS/ARRHYTHMIAS

- Electrolyte imbalances
- Hypoxia
- Medications

**Figure 5-1    Ectopic foci throughout the heart**

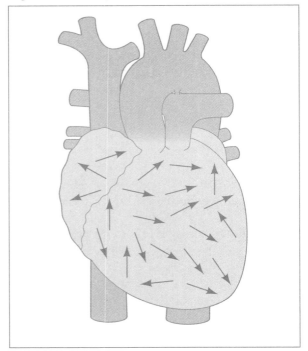

**Unifocal versus Multifocal**

**Unifocal:** an ectopic beat(s) and/or arrhythmia initiated from one abnormal foci within the heart.

**Multifocal:** an ectopic beat(s) and/or arrhythmia initiated from multiple abnormal foci within the heart.

*Source*: From *12-Lead ECG: The Art of Interpretation*, courtesy of Tomas B. Garcia, MD.

- Myocardial ischemia
- Pain
- Hypovolemia
- Hypervolemia
- Acidosis/Alkalosis
- Hypothermia
- An increase in sympathetic tone
- An imbalance between the sympathetic and parasympathetic systems
- An increase in the release of catecholamines (Lisbon & Fink, 2003; Packer, 2000)
- Restoration of coronary blood flow (reperfusion)

## TREATMENT FOR ECTOPIC BEATS/ARRHYTHMIAS

- Correct electrolyte imbalances, acid-base imbalances, and body temperature.
- Ensure adequate oxygenation and perfusion to the heart.
- Administer crystalloids and colloids as needed.
- Administer medications to slow and/or block arrhythmias as needed.
- Administer medications for pain control and sedation as needed.
- In emergency conditions, treat with electricity either through synchronized cardioversion, pacing, or defibrillation as per the American Heart Association guidelines (American Heart Association Guidelines, 2005).

# Normal Electrical Activity of the Heart

Please see Figure 6-1 for the electrical conduction system of the heart.

## SA NODE

The SA node is the natural pacemaker of the heart (see Figure 6-2). Under normal conditions the SA node assumes control of the electrical conduction system and acts as the "conductor" of the heart's electrical affairs (Packer, 2000). The SA node will try to suppress other foci that attempt to dominate or take over electrical conduction; however, the "automaticity center with the fastest rate" can overdrive the SA node and produce an ectopic beat(s) and/or arrythmia(s) (Dubin, 2000, p. 105).

- The intrinsic pacing rate of the SA node is 60 to 100.
- The heart prefers the natural pacemaker of the heart, the SA node, to assume pacemaker control.
- Under normal conditions the SA node fires and transmits an impulse that causes atrial contraction. This atrial contraction causes the blood to leave the atria and to enter the ventricle. This is known as "atrial kick" and can contribute up to 25–30% of the cardiac output (Eagan, 1996; Stewart & Vitello-Cicciu, 1996, p. 252).

> **Rhythms That Can Affect Atrial Kick**
>
> Atrial kick can be lost or minimized in atrial fibrillation, atrial flutter, and in junctional and ventricular rhythms.

**Figure 6-1   The electrical conduction system**

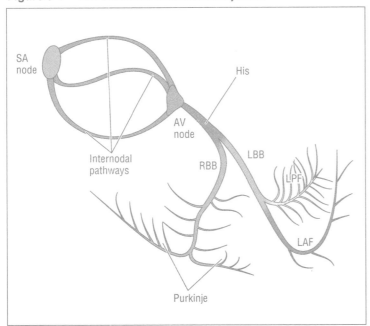

*Source*: From *12-Lead ECG: The Art of Interpretation*, courtesy of Tomas B. Garcia, MD.

**Figure 6-2   The SA node**

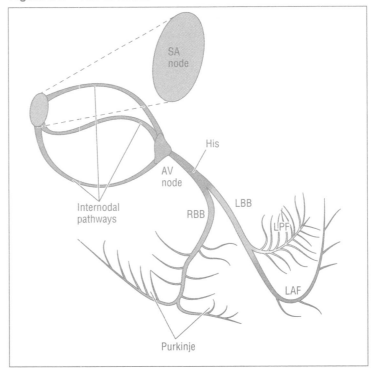

*Source*: From *12-Lead ECG: The Art of Interpretation*, courtesy of Tomas B. Garcia, MD.

## BACHMANN BUNDLE

Bachmann bundle is an accessory conduction pathway that transmits the electrical impulse from the right atria to the left atria.

## AV NODE

The AV node (see Figure 6-4) receives the electrical impulse from the SA node and acts as a conduit to transmit the impulse down to the ventricles. This is the only place in the electrical pathway where there is a slowing of the electrical impulse (Dubin, 2000). This slowing helps in the following ways:

- It allows the atria to complete their contractions and to fill the ventricles with blood.
- It inhibits some of the ectopic beats and/or arrhythmias that occur above the ventricle from being transmitted down to the ventricles because it is the only tissue that has decremented conduction properties, that is, the faster the electrical impulse is transmitted the slower it conducts.
- The AV node can assume pacemaker control of the heart if the SA fails to fire. The intrinsic pacing rate of the AV node is 40 to 60. When the AV node assumes pacemaker control of the heart, the rhythm is called a junctional rhythm (see Figure 6-5).

**Internodal, Interatrial, and Infranodal Tracts**

Please refer to Figure 6-3, the internodal pathway.

- The tracts that transmit the electrical impulse from the SA node to the AV node are known as the internodal pathways.
- The accessory conduction pathway that branches off one of the internodal tracts to transmit the electrical impulse across the atrial septum to the left atrium is referred to as the interatrial tract or Bachmann bundle (Allison, 1998).
- The tracts that transmit the electrical impulse from the AV node to the Purkinje network are referred to as the infranodal pathways.

**AV Node Protection**

Alcohol in excess, fatigue, cigarettes, fever, consumption of large amounts of caffeine, anxiety, infectious diseases, myocardial diseases, and pulmonary diseases may result in ectopic beats in the atria (Naccarelli, Willerson, & Blomqvist, 1995). Some of these ectopic beats in the atria can be very rapid. The AV node protects the patient from lethal ventricular arrhythmias by blocking or inhibiting some of these atrial ectopic beats from being conducted down to the ventricle. AV node protection, however, can be affected by drugs or diseases that alter the state of the AV node.

**Figure 6-3   The internodal pathway**

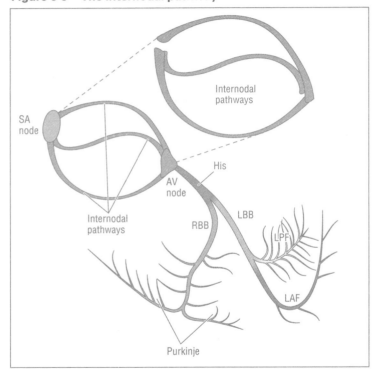

*Source*: From *12-Lead ECG: The Art of Interpretation*, courtesy of Tomas B. Garcia, MD.

**Figure 6-4   AV node**

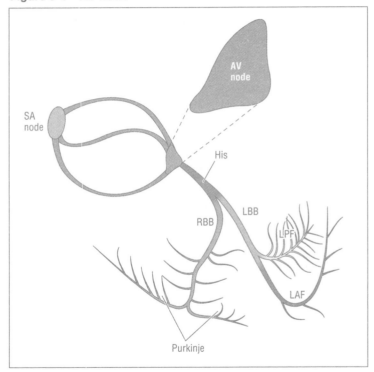

*Source*: From *12-Lead ECG: The Art of Interpretation*, courtesy of Tomas B. Garcia, MD.

- Some patients have abnormal pathways within and around the AV node that can override the normal electrical circuit. These abnormal pathways can transmit the electrical impulse speedily through the AV node or around the AV node in an antegrade and/or retrograde fashion. Two reentrant junctional tachyarrhythmias that use these abnormal pathways are atrioventricular nodal reentrant tachycardia (AVNRT) and AV bypass tachycardia (AVBT) (both will be covered in the rhythm section of the book).

---

**Antegrade and Retrograde**
- Antegrade conduction is the downward conduction of the electrical impulse. The impulse travels downward from the atria to the ventricles.
- Retrograde conduction is the backward or upward conduction of the electrical impulse. The impulse travels backward or upward from the AV node to the atria, or from the ventricle through the AV node or accessory pathway to the atria.

---

## THE BUNDLE OF HIS

The bundle of His (or His bundle; see Figure 6-6) is a "connective tissue sheet" that connects the upper and lower chambers of the heart (Cardiology, 2006, para. 3). It receives the electrical impulse from the AV node and speedily transmits the electrical impulse downward to the right and left bundle branches.

*Note:* An electrical impulse that is initiated lower on the His bundle or has a source of focus closer to the ventricle can produce a QRS complex that is wider than normal.

**Figure 6-5    Junctional rhythm**

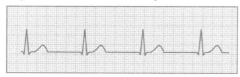

*Source*: Jackson, J. & Jackson, L. *Clinical nursing pocket guide*. Jones and Bartlett Publishers.

**Figure 6-6    The Bundle of His**

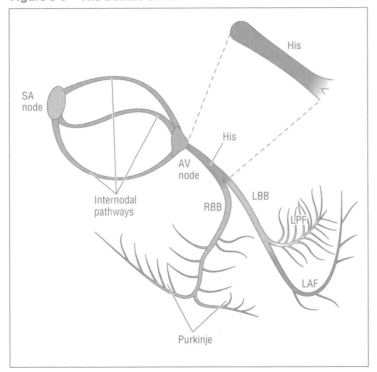

*Source*: From *12-Lead ECG: The Art of Interpretation*, courtesy of Tomas B. Garcia, MD.

**Figure 6-7    The Right Bundle Branch**

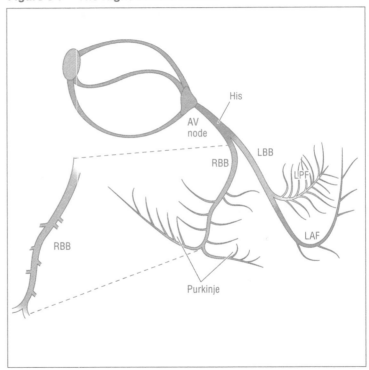

*Source*: From *12-Lead ECG: The Art of Interpretation*, courtesy of Tomas B. Garcia, MD.

## BUNDLE BRANCHES: RIGHT BUNDLE BRANCH AND LEFT BUNDLE BRANCH

The bundle branches transmit the electrical impulse to the right and the left ventricle.

### Right Bundle

The right bundle branch (see Figure 6-7) transmits the electrical impulse from the bundle of His down to the right ventricle.

> **Incomplete RBBB**
>
> An incomplete RBBB has the same QRS morphology as an RBBB, but the QRS is less than 0.12 sec or 120 ms (ACC/AHS/HRS, 2006; Wagner, 2008).

#### *Abnormal Condition of the Right Bundle: Right Bundle Branch Block*

A delay in the transmission of the electrical impulse down the right bundle is referred to as a right bundle branch block (RBBB; see Figure 6-8).

---

**Box 6-1    Assessment of a Right Bundle Branch Block**

- The QRS interval is greater than or equal to 0.12 sec or 120 ms (Garcia & Holtz, 2001).
- The QRS complex in $V_1$–$V_2$ leads (the right chest leads) can have an rsR′ or rSR′ configuration (a small initial R wave followed by a small or a large S wave, and a second R wave that is larger than the initial R wave). This configuration can look like rabbit ears (see Figure 6-9) (Garcia & Holtz, 2001).
- Wide, slurred S waves can be seen in $V_5$–$V_6$ and also in I and $aV_L$ (ACC/AHA/HRS, 2006; Garcia & Holtz, 2001; Ganz, 2003).
- Delayed onset of intrinsicoid deflection in $V_1$ and $V_2$ > 50 ms (or 0.05 sec). (Intrinsicoid deflection will be covered in the Right and Left Ventricular Hypertrophy section) (ACC/AHA/HRS, 2006; Garcia & Holtz, 2001; Ganz, 2003).
- Secondary ST-T wave changes can occur with an RBBB (Wagner, 2008).
- QRS complexes are predominately positive in lead $V_1$ (Sangrigoli & Hsia, 2002).
- Geiter (2003) writes that an assessment of a bundle branch block can be "accurately made using only $V_1$" (p. 32cc1).

---

Note: The R′ in a RBBB represents a delay in the depolarization of the right ventricle.

**Figure 6-8   Right bundle branch block**

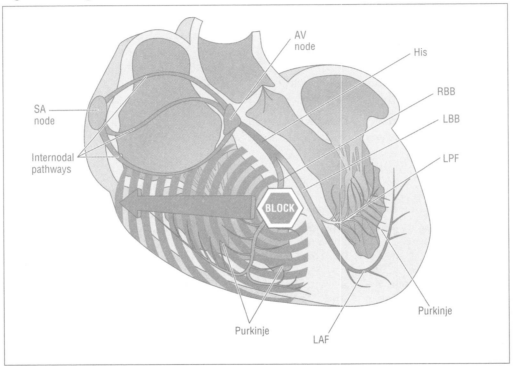

*Source*: From *12-Lead ECG: The Art of Interpretation*, courtesy of Tomas B. Garcia, MD.

## Other Considerations

- A RBBB can make it difficult to differentiate between supraventricular tachycardia (SVT) and ventricular tachycardia (VT) (Hebbar & Hueston, 2002).
- A new RBBB after an acute myocardial infarction (AMI) can be indicative of a "very large" area of myocardial ischemia/infarction (Wagner, Selvester, White, & Wagner, 1995, p. 234).

**Figure 6-9    The ECG and Right Bundle Branch Block**

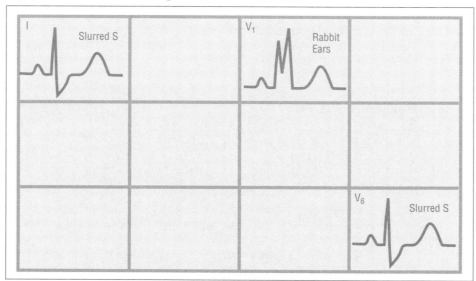

*Source*: From *12-Lead ECG: The Art of Interpretation*, courtesy of Tomas B. Garcia, MD.

- A RBBB combined with a left bundle branch block (LBBB) requires careful monitoring because it can lead to a "sudden occurrence of complete atrioventricular block" (Wagner et al., 1995, p. 234).
- A RBBB can make it difficult to assess the electrical axis of the heart.

## Left Bundle

The left bundle starts as one common bundle and then separates into two: the anterior and the posterior fascicle (see Figure 6-10). Some patients also have a middle fascicle. These fascicles transmit the electrical impulse from the bundle of His down to different areas of the left ventricle. The reason the left bundle needs more electrical circuits is because the muscle on the left side of the heart is bigger.

### *Abnormal Condition of the Left Bundle: Left Bundle Branch Block*
A delay in the transmission of the electrical impulse down the left common bundle is referred to as an LBBB (see Figure 6-10a).

---

**Box 6-2   Assessment of a Left Bundle Branch Block**

- The QRS interval is greater than or equal to 0.12 sec or 120 ms (Garcia & Holtz, 2001).
- rS or QS configurations can be seen in the right chest leads ($V_1$, $V_2$) (Wagner, 2008).
- The R waves are often wide and slurred or notched in I, a$V_L$, $V_5$, $V_6$ (Garcia & Holtz, 2001 & Ganz, 2003).
- ST and T wave deflections are opposite from the QRS complex, and the T wave is often inverted (ACC/AHA/HRS, 2006).
- There is a delayed onset of intrinsicoid deflection in 1, $V_5$, and $V_6$ > 60 ms or 0.06 sec (ACC/AHA/HRS, 2006, Ganz, 2003; Wagner, 2008).
- The QRS complex in leads I, $V_5$–$V_6$ (the left chest leads) have an rsR' pattern (a small initial R wave followed by a small S wave and a second R wave that is larger than the initial R wave) or RR' pattern (a large initial R wave followed by a second large R wave) (ACC/AHA/HRS, 2006).
- The QRS complex is negative in $V_1$. A large Q wave can be found in $V_1$ and a large R wave in $V_6$ (Geiter, 2003).

Note: The R' in a LBBB represents a delay in the depolarization of the left ventricle.

---

**Figure 6-10a    The Left Bundle Branch**

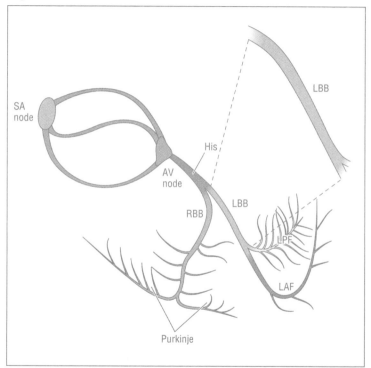

Source: From *12-Lead ECG: The Art of Interpretation*, courtesy of Tomas B. Garcia, MD.

**Figure 6-10    The Left Bundle Branch Block**

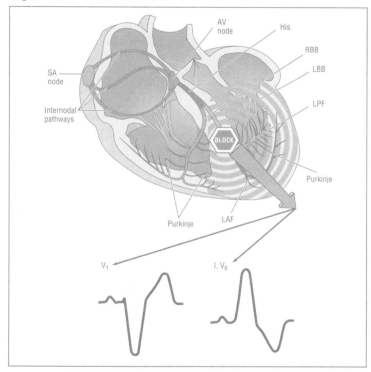

Source: From *12-Lead ECG: The Art of Interpretation*, courtesy of Tomas B. Garcia, MD.

**Fascicle**

A fascicle is a band or a bundle of fibers. In the heart this bundle of fibers includes the right bundle branch; the left bundle branch; the anterior, posterior, and middle fascicles; and the Purkinjes.

**Box 6-3  A Scoring System to Assist in Making the Diagnosis of an AMI in the presence of an LBBB**

- ST segment elevation > or equal to 1 mm that is concordant (in the same direction) with the QRS        5 pts.
- ST segment depression > or equal to 1 mm in leads $V_1$, $V_2$, or $V_3$ with a predominantly negative QRS        3 pts
- ST elevation > or equal to 5 mm in leads $V_1$ and $V_2$ discordant (in the opposite direction) with the QRS        2 pts

Note: Although this scoring system has a low sensitivity (Haywood, 2005), it offers to the clinician an optional tool to assist with risk stratification of patients presenting with an LBBB and AMI (Wong et al., 2005).

*Source*: Sgarbossa et al., 1996a; Sgarbossa et al., 1996b.

### Other Considerations

- A LBBB on a 12-lead EKG can make the diagnosis of an AMI difficult to determine (Murphy, 2000b; Vacek, 2002) because the LBBB can obscure the ST segments and the Q waves (Alpert, Thygesen, Antman, & Bassand, 2000). To assist in making the diagnosis when there is an LBBB, compare the patient's old EKG with the patient's new EKG (Haberl, 2002–2005).

- The scoring system in Box 6-3 can also be used to assist in making the diagnosis of an AMI in patients with an LBBB. A total score greater than or equal to 3 yields a "90%" specificity and an "88%" positive predictive value for an AMI (Bhatia & Kaul, 2007, p. 8; Edhouse, Brady, & Morris, 2002, para. 8–9; Sgarbossa et al., 1996a; Sgarbossa et al., 1996b).

- Patients with a new or presumably new LBBB who present with symptoms of an acute myocardial infarction, regardless of the algorithm score, are five times more likely to have an acute myocardial infarction and should be treated similarly to patients who present with an ST segment elevation myocardial infarction (Conover, 2003; National Guideline Clearinghouse, 1998–2008).

- A LBBB can make it difficult to differentiate between an SVT and ventricular tachycardia (Hebbar & Hueston, 2002).

- A new LBBB after an AMI can be indicative of a "very large" area of myocardial ischemia/infarction (Wagner et al., 1995, p. 234).

- A LBBB alternating with a right bundle branch block requires careful monitoring because it can lead to a "sudden occurrence of complete atrioventricular block" (Wagner et al., 1995, p. 234).

- A LBBB can make it difficult to assess the electrical axis of the heart.

## BRANCHES OFF OF THE LEFT BUNDLE: ANTERIOR, POSTERIOR, AND MIDDLE FASCICLE

The extra branches off of the left bundle assist in transmitting electrical signals to various areas of the left ventricle.

### Anterior Fascicle

The anterior fascicle (see Figure 6-11) transmits the electrical impulse to the "anterior superior endocardial surface of the left ventricle" (Stewart & Vitello-Cicciu, 1996, p. 252).

**Figure 6-11    Anterior fascicle**

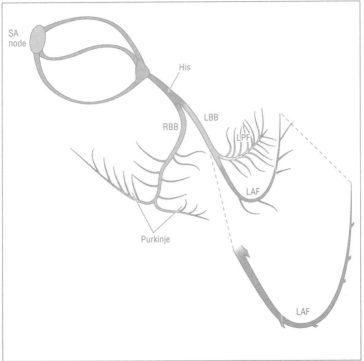

*Source*: From *12-Lead ECG: The Art of Interpretation*, courtesy of Tomas B. Garcia, MD.

## Posterior Fascicle

The posterior fascicle (see Figure 6-12) transmits the electrical impulse to the "posterior inferior region of the left ventricle's endocardial surface" (Stewart & Vitello-Cicciu, 1996, p. 252).

## Middle Fascicle

Some patients also have a third fascicle (Murphy, 2000a). This fascicle is called the left septal, middle, or median fascicle. It is found in 65% of people, and it transmits the electrical impulse to the interventricular septum (Arnsdorf, n.d.).

## ABNORMAL CONDITIONS OF THE FASCICLES: FASCICULAR BLOCKS

- A block of the anterior fascicle is referred to as an anterior hemiblock.
- A block of the posterior fascicle is referred to as a posterior hemiblock.
- A block of the right bundle branch along with the anterior or the posterior fascicle is called a bifasicular block.
- A block of the right bundle branch along with the anterior and posterior fascicle is called a third-degree heart block or complete heart block.
- A block of two fascicles and an intermittent block of the third fascicle is referred to as a type II second-degree heart block or Mobitz type II block.
- A block of the left common bundle before it branches into the anterior and the posterior fascicle is referred to as a left bundle branch block (refer back to Figure 6-10a).

**Box 6-4   Assessment of an Anterior Hemiblock (see Figure 6-13):**
- Left axis deviation
- Q wave in lead I
- Wide and/or deep S wave in lead III
- QRS interval is 0.10–0.12 sec or 100–120 ms
- Block is often associated with left coronary artery occlusions

**Box 6-5   Assessment of a Posterior Hemiblock (see Figure 6-14)**
- Right axis deviation
- Wide and deep S wave in lead I
- Q wave in lead III
- QRS interval is 0.10–0.12 sec or 100–120 ms
- Block is often associated with right coronary artery disease

**Figure 6-12   Posterior fascicle**

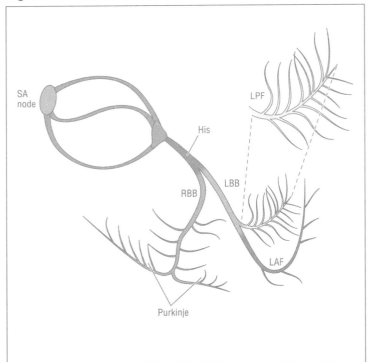

*Source*: From *12-Lead ECG: The Art of Interpretation*, courtesy of Tomas B. Garcia, MD.

**Figure 6-13   Anterior hemiblock**

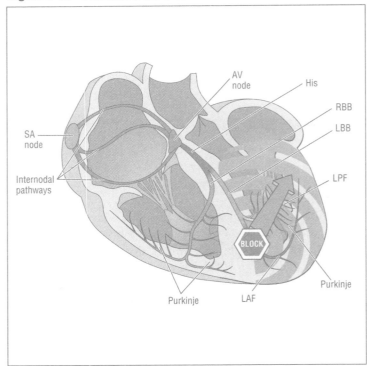

*Source*: From *12-Lead ECG: The Art of Interpretation*, courtesy of Tomas B. Garcia, MD.

## PURKINJE FIBERS

The Purkinje fibers (see Figure 6-15) transmit the electrical impulse from the ends of the bundle branches to the ventricles, from the endocardium to the epicardium, to initiate depolarization.

- The Purkinje fibers can assume pacemaker control of the heart if the SA node and the AV node fail to fire. The intrinsic rate of the Purkinje fibers is 20–40. When the Purkinje fibers in the ventricle assume pacemaker control of the heart, the rhythm is called an idioventricular rhythm (idio means "one's own"; see Figure 6-16).

**Three Layers of the Heart**

The three layers of the heart are as follows:

- Endocardium: The innermost layer of the heart wall.
- Myocardium: The middle and largest portion of the heart wall.
- Epicardium: The outer layer of the heart wall, which includes the visceral serous lining that surrounds the heart (Critical Care Nursing, 2004; Stewart & Vitello-Cicciu, 1996).

*Note:* A subendocardial myocardial infarction involves the endocardium, and a transmural myocardial infarction involves all three layers of the heart.

**Figure 6-14    Posterior hemiblock**

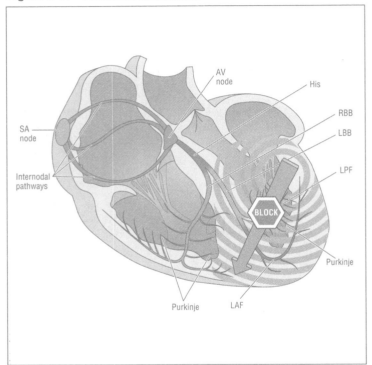

*Source*: From *12-Lead ECG: The Art of Interpretation*, courtesy of Tomas B. Garcia, MD.

**Figure 6-15    The Purkinje system**

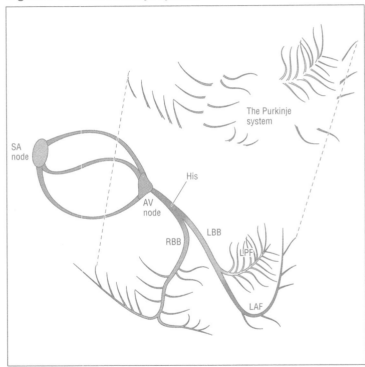

*Source*: From *12-Lead ECG: The Art of Interpretation*, courtesy of Tomas B. Garcia, MD.

**Figure 6-16  Idioventricular rhythm**

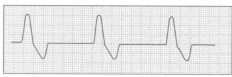

*Source*: Jackson, J. & Jackson, L. *Clinical nursing pocket guide*. Jones and Bartlett Publishers.

**Accelerated Idioventricular Rhythm**

When the idioventricular rhythm is faster than 40 beats per minute and less than 100 beats per minute, it is called an accelerated idioventricular rhythm (see Figure 6-17).

**Pacing Wires and the Endocardium and Epicardium**

- Pacing wires that are inserted transvenously pace the heart from the endocardium to the epicardium (from the inside of the heart to the outside of the heart). Example: Permanent pacemakers are inserted transvenously to pace patients who have cardiac conduction disturbances (Hayes, 1993; see Figure 6-18).
- Pacing wires that are loosely sutured to the outside of the heart, pace from the epicardium to the endocardium (from the outside of the heart to the inside of the heart). Example: Epicardial pacing wires that are sutured to the outside surface of the ventricular wall during cardiac surgery can be used to temporarily pace patients who have postoperative cardiac conduction disturbances (Hayes & Holmes, 1993; Stephens-Lesser, 2007).

**Figure 6-17   Accelerated idioventricular rhythm**

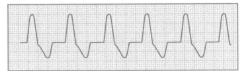

*Source*: Jackson, J. &Jackson, L. *Clinical nursing pocket guide*. Jones and Bartlett Publishers.

**Figure 6-18   Pacemaker wire in the endocardium**

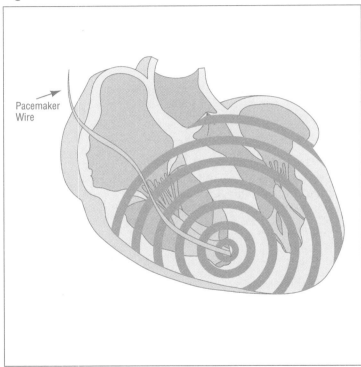

Pacemaker
Wire

*Source*: From *12-Lead ECG: The Art of Interpretation*, courtesy of Tomas B. Garcia, MD.

# Abnormal Electrical Conduction Pathways

## ABERRANT CONDUCTION

Aberrant conduction is an abnormal transmission of the electrical impulse from the atria to the ventricle. It occurs when a supraventricular (above the ventricles) electrical impulse is initiated prematurely, causing a temporary delay in transmission of the impulse through one of the bundle branches or the Purkinje fibers that have not completely repolarized from the previous electrical impulse. This delay in transmission of the impulse leads to the depolarization of one ventricle before the other and can produce a slightly widened QRS complex on the EKG that looks different from the normally conducted QRS complex (see Figure 7-1). Examples of terms often associated with aberrant conduction are as follows:

*Note:* An SVT with aberrant conduction that produces a slightly widened QRS complex can look like VT. (Refer to Tips to Assist in Differentiating SVT with Aberrant Conduction from VT in the rhythms section of the book.)

**Premature Beat**

A premature beat occurs when an electrical impulse is initiated too early in the electrical circuit of the heart.

- PAB with aberrant conduction is a premature atrial beat that is aberrantly conducted. (PAB is also know as a PAC, premature atrial complex.)
- PJB with aberrant conduction is a premature junctional beat that is aberrantly conducted. (PJB is also known as a PJC, premature junctional complex.)
- SVT with aberrant conduction is a supraventricular tachycardia that is aberrantly conducted.

**Figure 7-1   Rhythm strip with aberrant conduction**

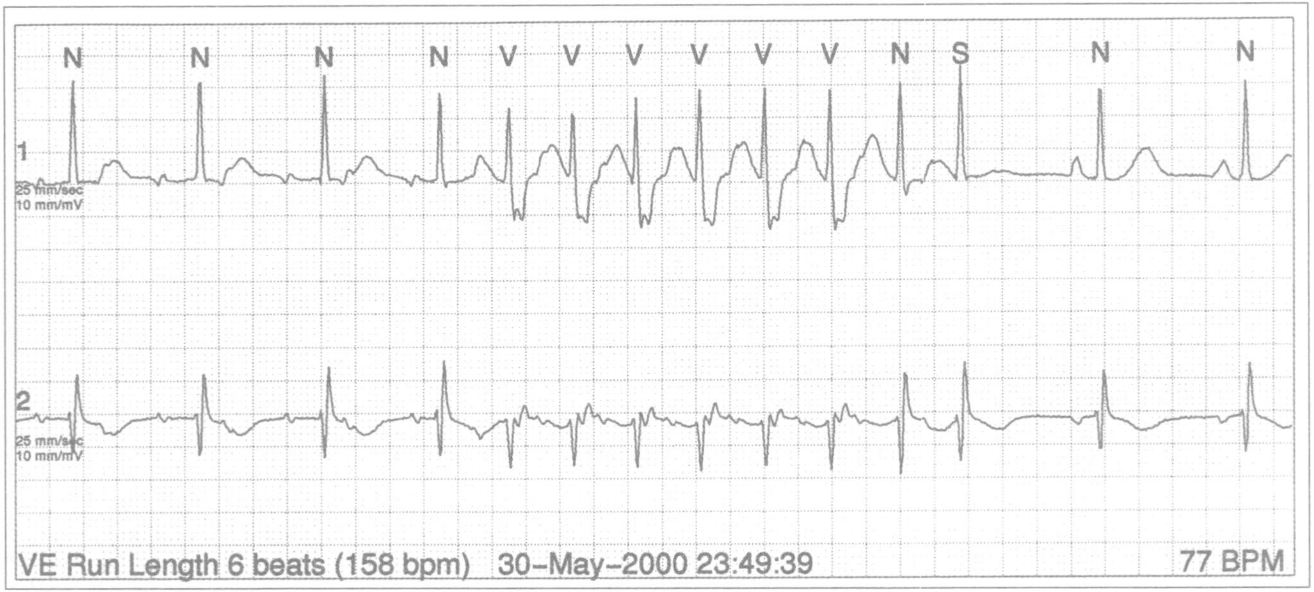

Source: Rosenthal, *Dx/Rx: Arrhythmias*. © 2008 by Jones and Bartlett Publishers.

## ACCESSORY PATHWAYS

Accessory pathways are abnormal pathways, or additional pathways, outside of the normal electrical circuit that can transmit the electrical impulse from the atria to the ventricles (antegrade conduction) or from the ventricles or the AV node to the atria (retro-

## ACCESSORY PATHWAYS

Accessory pathways are abnormal pathways, or additional pathways, outside of the normal electrical circuit that can transmit the electrical impulse from the atria to the ventricles (antegrade conduction) or from the ventricles or the AV node to the atria (retrograde conduction). An example of a rhythm that uses an accessory pathway is Wolff-Parkinson-White (WPW) syndrome.

### Wolff-Parkinson-White Syndrome

WPW occurs when an accessory AV conduction pathway (a pathway other than the AV node), historically called the Kent bundle, competes with the normal electrical circuit of the heart in the transmission of the electrical impulse from the atria to the ventricles (see Figure 7-2).

- The Kent bundle transmits the electrical impulse to a portion of the ventricles quicker than the AV node, resulting in a premature depolarization of a portion of the ventricles.
- This premature depolarization of the ventricles is seen as a delta wave on the EKG (see Figure 7-3).
- Other distinguishing characteristics of WPW include:
  - A shortened P-R interval
  - A wide QRS complex
  - Tachycardia associated with paroxysmal episodes of SVT, atrial fibrillation, and atrial flutter.
- Patients with WPW "carry the distinct risk of sudden cardiac death because of atrial fibrillation with a rapid rate" (Scheinman & Kaushik, 2003, p. 518).
- The treatment for WPW includes the following:
  - Patients with WPW should be referred to a cardiologist.
  - Medications that block conduction through the AV node should be avoided because this could increase transmission of the electrical impulse down the Kent bundle; for example, avoid adenosine, diltiazem, digoxin, and verapamil (American Heart Association Guidelines, 2005).

**Figure 7-2    The Bundle of Kent**

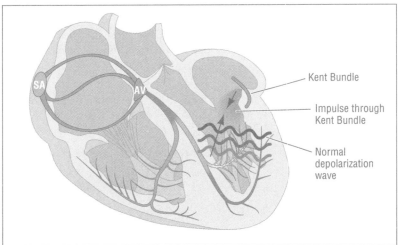

*Source*: From *12-Lead ECG: The Art of Interpretation*, courtesy of Tomas B. Garcia, MD.

**Figure 7-3   The Delta wave**

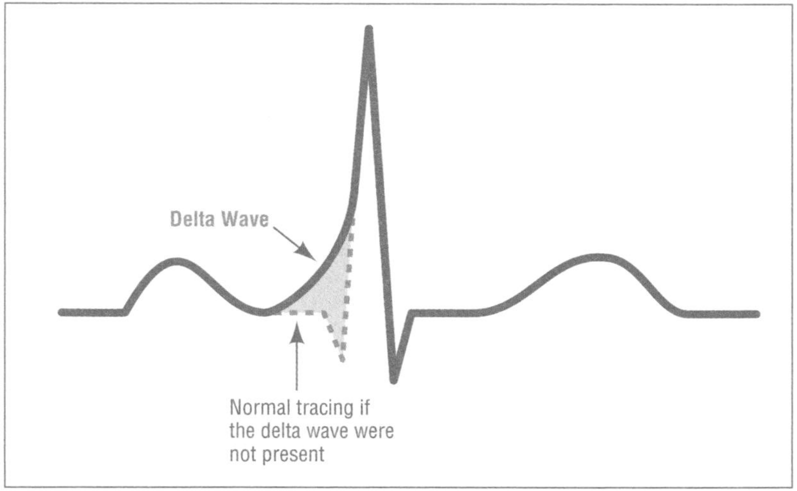

Delta Wave

Normal tracing if
the delta wave were
not present

*Source*: From *12-Lead ECG: The Art of Interpretation*, courtesy of Tomas B. Garcia, MD.

- Emergency treatment for WPW with atrial fibrillation includes the use of synchronized cardioversion, procainamide, and defibrillation if the patient's condition worsens.
- Long-term management includes ablation of the accessory pathway (Scheinman & Kaushik, 2003).

# SECTION 8

# Blood Supply to the Cardiac Conduction System

Please see Figure 8-1 for an illustration of the anterior view of the coronary arteries of the heart.

The electrical "components" of the heart and the coronary arteries that provide them with oxygen-rich blood are as follows:

* SA Node

The right coronary artery supplies blood to the SA node in 55–65% of the population (Packer, 2000). The left circumflex artery supplies blood to the SA node in 35–45% of the population (Packer, 2000).

* AV Node

The right coronary artery supplies blood to the AV node in 90% of the population (Packer, 2000). The left circumflex artery supplies blood to the AV node in 10% of the population (Stewart & Vitello-Cicciu, 1996).

* Bundle of His

The right coronary artery and the left anterior descending artery supply blood to the bundle of His (Packer, 2000).

> **Bradycardia and Blood Supply to the SA Node and the AV Node**
>
> Watch out for bradycardia in patients who have compromised blood supply to the SA node and/or the AV node.

**Figure 8-1    The coronary arteries of the heart**

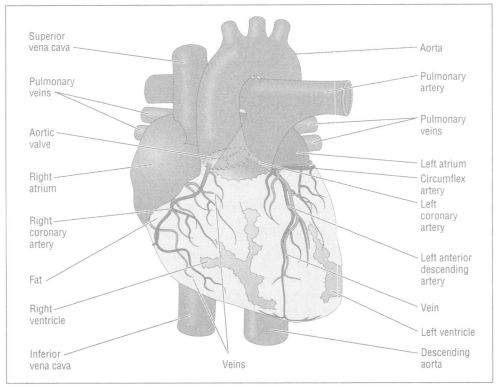

*Source*: From *12-Lead ECG: The Art of Interpretation*, courtesy of Tomas B. Garcia, MD.

- Right Bundle

The right coronary artery and the left anterior descending artery supply blood to the right bundle (Ferguson & Cox, 1995; Packer, 2000).

- Left Anterior Fascicle

The left anterior descending artery supplies blood to the left anterior fascicle (Ferguson & Cox, 1995; Packer, 2000).

- Left Middle Fascicle

The left anterior descending artery supplies blood to the left middle fascicle (Wagner et al., 1995).

- Left Posterior Fascicle

The right coronary artery, the left anterior descending artery, and the left circumflex supply blood to the left posterior fascicle (Ferguson & Cox, 1995; Packer, 2000; Stewart & Vitello-Cicciu, 1996).

# The Electrical Activity of the Heart and the EKG

Please see Figure 9-1 for a diagram of the EKG complex.

## P WAVE

The P wave reflects the contraction of the atria after the sinoatrial node transmits an electrical pulse (see Figure 9-2 and Figure 9-3).

**Figure 9-1    The ECG complex**

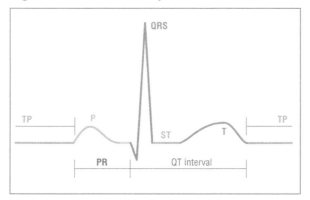

*Source*: From *12-Lead ECG: The Art of Interpretation*, courtesy of Tomas B. Garcia, MD.

**Figure 9-2    The P wave**

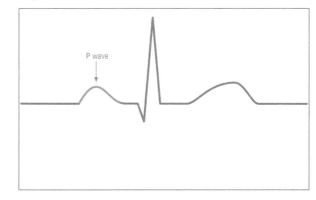

*Source*: From *12-Lead ECG: The Art of Interpretation*, courtesy of Tomas B. Garcia, MD.

**Figure 9-3   The SA node transmits an electrical impulse causing a P wave on the ECG**

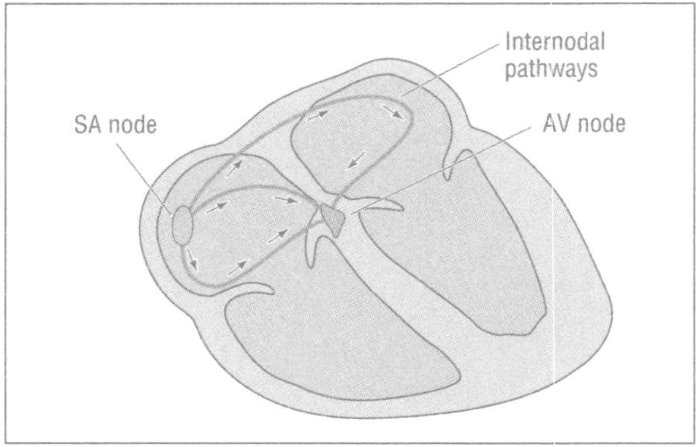

*Source*: From *12-Lead ECG: The Art of Interpretation*, courtesy of Tomas B. Garcia, MD.

## Normal Conditions of P the Wave

- The duration of the P wave (measured from the beginning of the P wave to the end of the P wave) is normally 0.08 to 0.11 sec or 80 to 110 ms.
- The height of the P wave is normally less than 2.5mm. (0.25mV).

**Monophasic versus Diphasic**

Monophasic: The contour of the EKG complex has one phase that is either entirely positive or entirely negative.

Diphasic: The contour of the EKG complex has two phases that include a positive and a negative, often referred to as double humped.

- P waves should be monophasic and uniform in size and shape.
- P waves should precede each QRS complex, that is, one P wave should be associated with one QRS complex.

## Abnormal Conditions of P Waves

- P waves are not found on the EKG complex.
- A P wave does not precede each QRS complex.
- The P waves do not correspond with atrial contraction, i.e., electrical activity but no mechanical activity.
- The P waves are different in shape and size from the normal sinus P wave.
  - A P wave that is diphasic and has a height greater than or equal to 2.5 mm (0.25 mV) is associated with right atrial enlargement.
  - A P wave that is diphasic and has a duration greater than or equal to 120 ms or 0.12 sec is associated with left atrial enlargement. Left atrial enlargement can increase the risk of atrial tachyarrhythmias, embolisms, and left atrial electromechanical dysfunction (Ariyarajah, Mercado, Apiyasawat, Puri, & Spodick, 2005).

# P-R INTERVAL

The P-R interval reflects the interval of time from the beginning of the P wave to the beginning of the QRS complex as the electrical impulse travels from the sinoatrial node (SA node), through the atrioventricular node (AV node), down the His bundle, the bundle branches, and the Purkinje fibers (see Figure 9-4).

## Normal Condition of the P-R Interval

The normal P-R interval is 0.12–0.20 sec or 120–200 ms and is level with the isoelectric line (see Figure 9-5).

**Figure 9-4 The PR interval as it relates to the electrical conduction system**

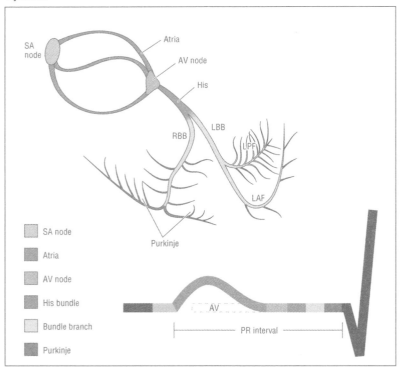

*Source*: From *12-Lead ECG: The Art of Interpretation*, courtesy of Tomas B. Garcia, MD.

**Figure 9-5 Normal PR interval**

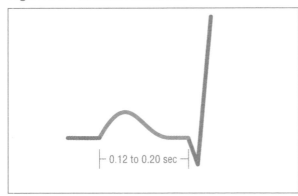

*Source*: From *12-Lead ECG: The Art of Interpretation*, courtesy of Tomas B. Garcia, MD.

## Abnormal Conditions of the P-R Interval

- A prolonged P-R interval is > 0.20 sec or 200 ms.
  - A prolonged P-R interval suggests that there may be interference in transmission of the electrical impulses through the atria, the AV node, the bundle of His, and/or the Purkinje fibers. (Interference at the AV node is the most common cause.)
  - Slowed conduction of the electrical impulses through the AV node is the most common cause of first degree heart blocks and Type 1 second degree heart blocks (Wenckebach).
- A shortened P-R interval is < 0.12 sec or 120 ms (see Figure 9-6).
  - Shortened P-R intervals can be found in preexcitation rhythms such as Wolff-Parkinson-White (WPW) syndrome and Lown-Ganong-Levine syndrome.
  - Shortened P-R intervals can also be associated with the use of catecholamines, enhanced atrioventricular nodal conduction, pregnancy, and childhood/adolescence (Ganz, 2003, p. 178).
- A P-R interval that is above or below the isoelectric line.
  - P-R segment depression in leads II, III, and aV$_F$, and P-R segment elevation in lead aV$_R$, may be seen in acute pericarditis (Nishimura & Kidd, 2003).

**The Isoelectric Line**

The isoelectric line is the horizontal line on the EKG that serves as a baseline for measurement of cardiac electrical activity. The P-R interval and/or the T-P interval (the interval of time from the end of the T wave to the beginning of the P wave) can serve as a guide in identifying the isoelectric line.

*Note:* Lown-Ganong-Levine syndrome is a preexcitation syndrome associated with " 'enhanced AV nodal conduction' and SVT" (Ganz, 2003, p. 178). EKG characteristics include a shortened P-R interval without the prescence of a delta wave because ventricular activation is normal.

**Figure 9-6    Shortened PR interval**

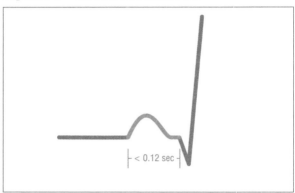

*Source*: From *12-Lead ECG: The Art of Interpretation*, courtesy of Tomas B. Garcia, MD.

## QRS COMPLEX

The QRS complex reflects the contraction of the ventricle after the Purkinje fibers transmit an electrical impulse. It is measured from the beginning of the Q to the end of the S (see Figures 9-7 and 9-8).

### Normal Conditions of the QRS Complex

- A normal QRS complex is 0.08 to < 0.12 sec or 80 to < 120 ms (see Figures 9-7 and 9-8).
  - A complex equal to or greater than 0.12 sec or 120 ms is a characteristic of an abnormally wide QRS complex (ACC/AHA/HRS, 2006; Scheinman & Kaushik, 2003).

**Figure 9-7   The QRS complex**

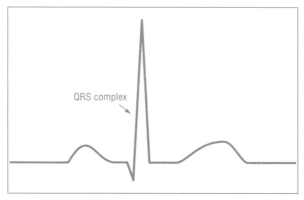

*Source*: From *12-Lead ECG: The Art of Interpretation*, courtesy of Tomas B. Garcia, MD.

**Figure 9-8   Measuring the QRS complex**

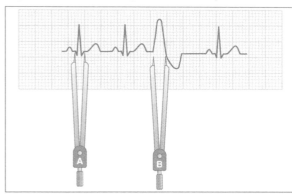

*Source*: From *12-Lead ECG: The Art of Interpretation*, courtesy of Tomas B. Garcia, MD.

- A QRS complex should be seen after every P wave.
- QRS complexes should be uniform in size and shape.

## Abnormal Conditions of the QRS Complex

- QRS complexes are not found on the EKG complex.
- A QRS complex is not found after every P wave.
- The QRS complex is asynchronous from the P wave.
- The QRS complex does not correspond with ventricular contraction, i.e., electrical activity but no mechanical activity.

- The QRS complex is equal to or greater than 0.12 sec or 120 ms.
  - Wide QRS complexes can be seen in bundle branch blocks, ventricular rhythms, and supraventricular tachycardias with aberrant conduction.
- A QRS complex contains a pathologic Q wave (see Figure 9-9).
- The QRS complex is different in shape and size from the normal sinus QRS
  - Ventricular hypertrophy
    - Ventricular hypertrophy occurs as the ventricular wall(s) become enlarged in an effort to compensate

**Figure 9-9   A pathologic Q wave**

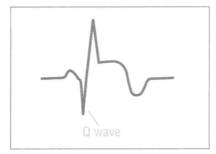

Q wave

*Source*: Porter, W. *Porter's pocket guide to emergency and critical care.* Jones and Bartlett Publishers.

**Pathologic Q Wave and Myocardial Infarction**

- A Q wave occurs when an injury is not fixed in a timely fashion and there is death to some portion or portions of the myocardium.
- A Q wave with a width greater than or equal to 0.04 sec and/or a height greater than or equal to one-quarter the amplitude of the R wave in at least two contiguous leads can be pathologic and indicative of a myocardial infarction (ACC/AHA/HRS, 2006).
- There is a high mortality rate for patients who develop Q waves early in acute myocardial infarction (Walling, 2006).

**Q, R, and S Waves**

It is important to note that not every QRS complex will have all three components, that is, the Q, the R, and the S.

- The Q wave is the first negative deflection of the QRS complex.
  - A normal Q wave is small and < 0.02-0.03 sec, except in leads III and $aV_R$, where any size of the Q wave is normal (Wagner & Lim, 2008a).
  - Any Q waves found in leads $V_1$, $V_2$, or $V_3$ are abnormal (Wagner & Lim, 2008a).
  - An absence of Q waves in leads $V_5$ and $V_6$ is abnormal (Wagner & Lim, 2008a).
- The R wave is the first positive deflection of the QRS complex.
- The S wave is the second negative deflection after the R wave (Homoud, 2008).

or adapt to a chronic volume overload (an increase in preload) or a chronic pressure overload (an increase in afterload) (Wagner & Lim, 2008b).

- This pressure overload causes the ventricle(s) to work harder which results in an increase in size of the myocardial fibers and thickness of the ventricular wall(s).
- Ventricular hypertrophy can occur on the right side (right ventricular hypertrophy), the left side (left ventricular hypertrophy), or both sides (biventricular hypertrophy).

---

**Non-Q-Wave Myocardial Infarction**

A myocardial infarction (MI) that does not produce a pathologic Q wave on the EKG is called a non-Q-wave MI.

- Non-Q-wave myocardial infarctions are often referred to as subendocardial infarctions.
- These patients should be monitored closely because the area of injury often starts small but can extend to other portions of the heart.
- EKG characteristics can include T wave inversion without ST segment elevation or without pathologic Q waves.
- To assist in the identification of a non-Q-wave MI, assess the patient's signs and symptoms, obtain a patient history, electrocardiogram, and cardiac biochemical markers, such as cardiac troponin and CPK-MB (creatine phosphokinase-MB form). Additional clinical studies such as an echocardiogram can also be useful.

---

**Right Ventricular Hypertropy**

- EKG characteristics of right ventricular hypertrophy must include a QRS duration < 0.12 sec or 120 ms and at least one other criteria (ACC/AHA/HRS, 2006, p. 2551; Ganz 2003; Wagner & Lim, 2008b):
  - Right axis deviation (greater than or equal to 110°)
  - Prominent R wave and small S wave in $V_1$
  - R/S ratio in $V_1$ > 1 or R/S ratio in $V_5$ or $V_6$ less than or equal to 1 (see Figure 9-23a).
  - R wave in $V_1$ > or equal to 7 mm
  - R wave in $V_1$ + S wave in $V_5$ or $V_6$ greater than 10.5 mm
  - $rSR^1$ in $V_1$ with $R^1$ greater than 10 mm
  - qR complex in $V_1$
  - Abnormal R wave progression
- Secondary ST-T wave changes in right precordial leads ($V_1$ and $V_2$) (often an inverted T wave in $V_1$–$V_2$)
- Right atrial abnormality
- Onset of intrinsicoid deflection in $V_1$ between 0.035 and 0.055 sec

## Left Ventricular Hypertrophy

The EKG characteristics of left ventricular hypertrophy include the use of several criteria, such as Sokolow-Lyon voltage, Cornell voltage, Cornell product, and Romhilt-Estes scoring system (ACC/AHA/HRS, 2006, p. 2551; Ganz, 2003, p. 186).

- Sokolow-Lyon voltage
  - S wave in $V_1$ + R wave in $V_5$ or $V_6$ > 35 mm or 3.5 mV or R wave in $aV_L$ > or equal to 11 mm or 1.1 mV
- Cornell voltage
  - R wave in $aV_L$ + S wave in $V_3$ > 20 mm or 2 mV in women or > 28 mm or 2.8 mV in males
- Cornell product
  - Cornell voltage X QRS duration > 2440 ms (in women, 6 mm is added to the Cornell voltage)
- Romhilt-Estes scoring system: LVH is likely with 4 points or more; LVH is present with 5 points or more. (ACC/AHA/HRS, 2006, p. 2551; Ganz, 2003):
  - Amplitude of the R wave or S wave in any limb lead > 2.0 mV or Amplitude of the S wave in $V_1$ or $V_2$ > 3.0 mV or Amplitude of the R wave in $V_5$ or $V_6$ > 3.0 mV      (3 points)
  - ST segment changes with or without   (1 or 2 points) digitalis
  - Left atrial abnormality      (3 points)
  - Left axis deviation (-30 degrees or more)   (2 points)
  - QRS duration > 90 ms      (1 point)
  - Intrinsicoid deflection in $V_5$ or $V_6$ =      (1 point) 0.05 to 0.07 sec

## Intrinsicoid Deflection

Intrinsicoid deflection (see Figure 9-10) reflects the period of the time that is required to transmit the electrical impulse from the endocardium (the inner layer of the heart) to the epicardium (the outer layer of the heart). It is measured from the beginning of the Q wave or the earliest R wave to the peak of the R wave.

- $V_1$ or $V_2$ is used to measure the intrinsicoid deflection for the right ventricle (normal upper limit is 0.035 sec).
- $V_5$ or $V_6$ is used to measure the intrinsicoid deflection for the left ventricle (normal upper limit is 0.045 sec).
- Any condition that would slow the transmission of the electrical impulse from the endocardium to the epicardium would increase the intrinsicoid deflection. Ventricular hypertrophy is one condition that would increase the intrinsicoid deflection (Wagner & Lim, 2008b).

- Causes of right ventricular hypertrophy include pulmonary embolism, pulmonary hypertension, valvular disease, congenital heart disease, heart failure, and myocardial infarction (Solomon, 2003).
- Causes of left ventricular hypertrophy include aortic stenosis, systemic hypertension, and idiopathic causes.

## ST SEGMENT

The ST segment reflects the period of time from the end of ventricular depolarization to the beginning of ventricular repolarization. The ST segment is measured at the J point.

### Normal Conditions and Assessment of the ST Segment

- The ST segment is measured relative to the P-R interval or the T-P interval (T wave to the P wave) (Nair & Glancy, 2002). The P-R and T-P intervals serve as a guide in identifying the isoelectric line. The P-R interval may be a better choice in tachyarrhythmias because the T-P interval may be difficult to find (Flanders, 2007). (Please refer to Figure 9-13.)
- ST segments should be horizontal, flat, and level with the isoelectric line on the rhythm strip.
- It is recommended to assess the ST segment in a supine position with the head of the bed no greater than 30–45 degrees. Assessing the ST segment in this position avoids misdiagnoses that are associated with patient repositioning (Drew, 2002; Drew & Krucoff, 1999; Drew, Pelter, Adams, & Wung, 1998; Flanders, 2007).
- A small percentage of healthy patients have ST segment depression (1–2%) (Ganz, 2003).
- It is difficult to assess ST segment changes with a left bundle branch block (Flanders, 2007) and with accelerated rhythms, such as accelerated idioventricular rhythm (Drew & Krucoff, 1999).
- The assessment of ST segments can assist in predicting if a patient will be successful in weaning from mechanical ventilation (Flanders, 2007).

**Strain Pattern and Ventricular Hypertrophy**

Please see Figure 9-11 for strain pattern and the ST segment.

- A strain pattern may be seen with marked hypertrophy and severe overload of one or both of the ventricles.
- Patients with ventricular strain have a higher morbidity rate and a higher incidence of adverse outcomes (Salles, Cardoso, Noqueira, Bloch, & Muxfeldt, 2006).
- ECG characteristics include:
  - An increase in the amplitude of the QRS complex
  - ST segment depression in I $aV_L$, $V_5$, and $V_6$; (Adams-Hamoda, Caldwell, Stotts, & Drew, 2003)
  - ST segments humped upward in the middle
  - Flipped, asymmetric T waves (Adams-Hamoda, et al., 2003)

**Figure 9-10    Intrinsicoid deflection**

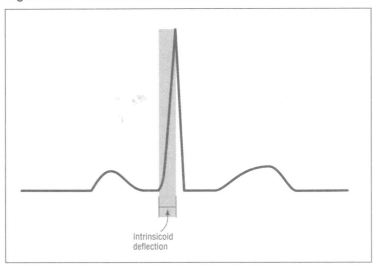

*Source*: From *Arrythmia Recognition: The Art of Interpretation*, courtesy of Tomas B. Garcia, MD and Geoffrey T. Miller, NREMT-P.

> *Note:* Intrinsicoid deflection is very helpful when trying to determine if a wide complex tachycardia is supraventricular tachycardia with aberrancy or ventricular tachycardia.

**Figure 9-11    Strain pattern and the ST segment**

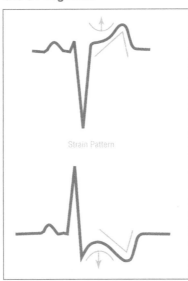

*Source*: From *12-Lead ECG: The Art of Interpretation*, courtesy of Tomas B. Garcia, MD.

**Figure 9-12    The J point & the ST segment**

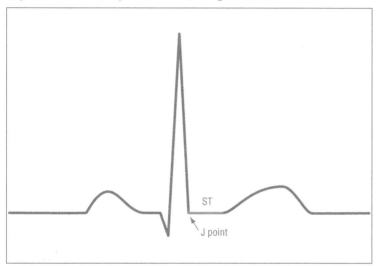

*Source*: From *12-Lead ECG: The Art of Interpretation*, courtesy of Tomas B. Garcia, MD.

**Figure 9-13    The isoelectric line & the ST segment**

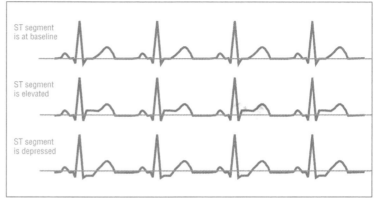

*Source*: From *12-Lead ECG: The Art of Interpretation*, courtesy of Tomas B. Garcia, MD.

**The J Point**

The J point is the point at which the end of the QRS complex meets the beginning of the ST segment. ST segments should be measured at the J point (ACC Clinical Data Standards, 2001; Thygesen, Alpert, & White, 2007). (Please refer to Figure 9-12.)

**Abnormal Conditions of the ST Segment**

## ST SEGMENT ELEVATION

(See Figure 9-14).

---

**The Contiguous Leads of the EKG**

Contiguous leads are as follows:

- Anterior: $V_1$, $V_2$, $V_3$, $V_4$, $V_5$, $V_6$
- Inferior: II, III, $aV_F$
- Lateral : I, $aV_L$

Courtesy of Thygesen, Alpert, & White, (2007).

---

**ST-segment Assessment Markers of an ST-segment elevation myocardial infarction (STEMI)**

EKG assessment markers that can assist with the classification of an ST-segment elevation myocardial infarction (STEMI) are as follows:

- A new or presumed new ST segment elevation that is greater than or equal to 1 mm or 0.1 mV at the J point in two contiguous precordial leads or two or more adjacent limb leads
- A new or presumed new ST segment elevation that is greater than or equal to 2 mm or 0.2 mV in men and greater than or equal to 1.5 mm or 0.15 mV in women in leads $V_1$–$V_3$ in the absence of a left bundle branch block and left ventricular hypertrophy.

Courtesy of Thygesen, Alpert, & White, (2007).

---

**Figure 9-14    ST segment elevation**

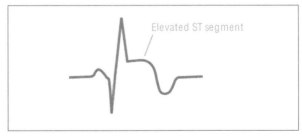

Elevated ST segment

*Source*: Porter, W. *Porter's pocket guide to emergency and critical care*. Jones and Bartlett Publishers.

## Myocardial Injury and ST Segment Elevation

- ST segment elevation associated with myocardial injury is an acute process caused by a total occlusion of one or more of the coronary arteries. The occlusion of the coronary artery (s) can lead to transmural damage of the heart if left untreated. Consequently, it is essential that ST segment elevation be treated immediately, by restoring and maintaining blood flow through the coronary artery (s), to preserve as much of the myocardium as possible (Homoud, 2008; Klabunde, 1999–2007).
- ST segment elevation can be referred to as "supply-related ischemia" (Booker, et al., 2003, p. 509), that is, ischemia induced when oxygen supply does not meet oxygen demand.
- The ST segment in acute coronary syndrome is convex or dome-shaped and can look like a tombstone (see Figure 9-15).

**Figure 9-15    ST segment tombstones**

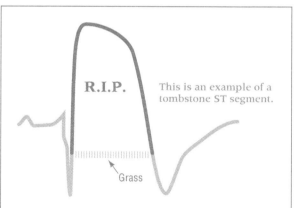

*Source*: From *12-Lead ECG: The Art of Interpretation*, courtesy of Tomas B. Garcia, MD.

- ST segment elevation can occur within the first minutes of an acute myocardial infarction and can persist hours to days (McAvoy, 2004).
- Typically, in patients who are having an acute myocardial infarction, there is ST segment elevation in the leads that "take a picture" of the injured region of the heart, and reciprocal changes in the leads that mirror the injured region of the heart.

### Reciprocal Changes

Reciprocal changes occur as the noninjured area (s) of the myocardium compensates for the injured area (s). Reciprocal changes can include:

- Qs become Rs.
- Elevated ST segments become depressed ST segments.
- Inverted T waves become upright T waves.

> *Note:* Reciprocal changes can make it difficult to determine if a depressed ST segment is from ischemia or from an acute injury.

**Table 9-1   Reciprocal Changes and the EKG**

| ST Segment Elevation | ST Segment Depression (Reciprocal Changes) |
| --- | --- |
| Anterior ($V_1$–$V_4$) | Inferior (II, III, $aV_F$) |
| Lateral (I, $aV_L$, $V_5$, $V_6$) | Inferior (II, III, $aV_F$) |
| Inferior (II, III, $aV_F$) | Lateral and anterior (I, $aV_L$, $V_1$–$V_6$) |
| Posterior ($V_1$–$V_3$) | Anterior ($V_1$–$V_3$) |

## Other Conditions Associated with ST Segment Elevation Include

- Head injury/subarachnoid hemorrhage
- Underlying ST segment elevations that can disappear in therapeutic hypothermia and reappear when the patient is rewarmed (Tan & Meregalli, 2007)
- Hyperthyroidism
- Hyperkalemia
- Propofol infusion syndrome that causes cardiac instability
  - An adverse reaction to a propofol infusion can cause cardiac instability. ST segment elevation in leads $V_1$–$V_3$ may be the first sign that the cardiac system has been compromised by a propofol infusion (Zaccheo & Bucher, 2008).
- Left bundle branch block
- Left ventricular hypertrophy
- Ventricular aneurysm
- Coronary vasospasm
- Normal variants
  - Ninety percent of healthy young men can have concave ST segment elevations that are 1–3 mm or 0.1–0.3 mV, "most marked in $V_2$" (Bhatia & Kaul, 2007, p. 8).
- Early repolarization
  - A normal and benign variant found on the EKGs of athletes and young black men.
  - In some patients, however, early repolarization has been found to be associated with sudden cardiac arrest (Haissaguerre, Derval, Sacher, Jesel, Deisenhofer, Roy, et al., 2008).
- Acute Pericarditis
  - Is an inflammation of the pericardium.
- Brugada syndrome

*Note:* Propofol (Diprivan) is a short-acting sedative-hypnotic agent used for general anesthesia or sedation.

### Early Repolarization, Acute Pericarditis, and ST segment elevation

ST segment elevation is a characteristic feature of the EKG in early repolarization and acute pericarditis. To assist in determining if the ST segment elevation is the result of a myocardial injury, early repolarization, or acute percardititis obtain a patient history, perform a physical examination, and assess the EKG.

### Brugada Syndrome and ST Segment Elevation

- Brugada syndrome is an inherited disorder that disrupts the normal electrical circuit of the heart and predisposes the patient to a high risk of sudden death.
- Brugada syndrome occurs more frequently in people of Asian ancestry (US National Library of Medicine, 2008).
- Brugada syndrome is 8 to 10 times more common in men than in women (US National Library of Medicine, 2008).
- Fifteen percent of patients have an abnormality in the SCN5A gene. This abnormality reduces the flow of sodium ions into the cells during the action potential, increasing the patient's risk of recurrent ventricular tachycardia or ventricular fibrillation (Scheinman & Kaushik, 2003; US National Library of Medicine, 2008).
- In patients without an abnormality in the SCN5A gene, the cause of the syndrome is unknown but may be attributed to certain drugs and certain electrolyte imbalances (US National Library of Medicine, 2008).
- To assist in identifying patients with Brugada syndrome, be aware of the EKG patterns associated with the condition and obtain a thorough patient history and family history.
- Brugada syndrome is "the most common cause of sudden cardiac death in patients with a structurally normal heart" (Sovari, Prasun, & Kocheril, 2007, para. 4).
- Amiodarone has been found to be effective in emergency situations, but the primary treatment is an implantable cardioverter defibrillator to prevent sudden cardiac death (Sovari, et al., 2007).

> **Characteristic EKG Findings Associated with Brugada Syndrome.**
> - Right bundle branch block, complete or incomplete.
> - ST segment elevation in leads $V_1$–$V_3$ at rest. The ST segment, however, can vary over time and can be affected by certain drugs, fever, exercise, and changes in heart rate (Brugada syndrome, n.d.).

**Characteristic EKG Findings Associated with Early Repolarization and Acute Pericarditis (Bhatia & Kaul, 2007; Conover, 2003; Goyle & Walling, 2002; Marinella, 1998):**

*ST SEGMENTS*
- ST segments are concave upward (saddle shaped), elevated from 1–4 mm, and resemble a fishhook pattern or a smile (see Figure 9-16) (Adams-Hamoda, et al., 2003; Nishimura & Kidd, 2003; Pelter & Carey, 2007).
- In acute pericarditis there is a greater degree of ST segment elevation when compared to the ST segment associated with early repolarization.
- There are no reciprocal changes associated with the elevated ST segments.
- ST segment elevations occur in the precordial leads. In acute pericarditis there is widespread ST segment elevation in the precordial and the limb leads (Wagner & Wang, 2008b).
- The ST/T ratio in lead $V_6$ > 0.25 mm is highly suggestive for acute pericarditis:
  - Obtain the ratio in lead $V_6$ by using the elevation of the ST segment in millimeters and the height of the T wave in millimeters. *Example: If the ST segment is 2 mm and the T wave is 5 mm in lead $V_6$ the ST/T ratio would be 0.40 mm which would be highly suggestive for acute pericarditis.*

*J POINTS*
- J points are elevated and can be notched.

*T WAVES*
- T waves are upright. In acute pericarditis T waves can become flat and inverted as the the ST segment returns to baseline.

*ANORMAL Q WAVES*
- There are no abnormal Q waves unless the patient has had a myocardial infarction.

*PR INTERVALS*
- P-R depression is usually not found in early repolarization but is common in acute pericarditis.

**Figure 9-16   ST segment, pericarditis, and early repolarization**

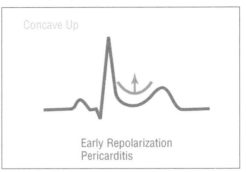

*Source*: From *12-Lead ECG: The Art of Interpretation*, courtesy of Tomas B. Garcia, MD.

To assist in differentiating between Brugada syndrome and acute coronary syndrome, look for the criteria shown in Table 9-2 (Riezebos, Man, Patterson, & Ruiter, 2007).

## ST SEGMENT DEPRESSION

Please see Figure 9-17 for ST segment depression.

## MYOCARDIAL INJURY OR ISCHEMIA AND ST SEGMENT DEPRESSION

- ST segment depression can reflect myocardial injury or myocardial ischemia.
- ST segment depression in leads $V_1$ through $V_3$ without ST segment elevation in any other leads can reflect posterior (infer-obasal) ischemia or infarction (Alpert, et al., 2000).

**Figure 9-17    ST segment depression**

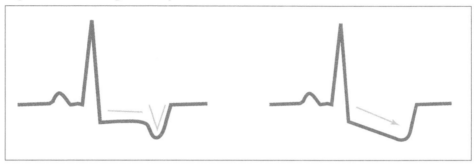

*Source*: From *12-Lead ECG: The Art of Interpretation*, courtesy of Tomas B. Garcia, MD.

**Table 9-2    A Comparison of Acute Coronary Syndrome and Brugada Syndrome**

| Acute Coronary Syndrome | Brugada Syndrome |
|---|---|
| ST segments are convex | ST segments are coved |
| Reciprocal ST depression | No reciprocal ST depression |
| Structural abnormalities | No structural abnormalities |
| Often symptomatic | Often asymptomatic and undiagnosed until the patient develops a polymorphic ventricular tachycardia, ventricular fibrillation, syncope, or nocturnal agonal respirations |

- ST segment depression can be seen in the leads that are reciprocal to the area of the heart that has been damaged.
- ST segment depression is referred to as "demand-related ischemia" (Booker, et al., 2003, p. 509), that is, ischemia induced when there is an increase in oxygen demand (oxygen consumption) but an inadequate flow of blood to meet the increased demand.

## Other Conditions Associated with ST Segment Depression Include

(Adams-Hamoda, et al., 2003; Casey, Morrissey, & Nolan, 1996; Diepenbrock, 2004)

- Hypokalemia
- Exercise
- Hypomagnesemia
- Normal variants
- Suctioning
- Hypothermia
- Hyperventilation
- Left ventricular hypertrophy
- Head injury/subarachnoid hemorrhage
- Digitalis

---

**ST-segment Assessment Marker of a Non-ST-segment elevation myocardial infarction (NSTEMI).**

An EKG assessment marker that can assist with the classification of a Non-ST-segment elevation myocardial infarction (NSTEMI) is as follows:

- ST depression that is new or downsloping and is greater than or equal to 0.5 mm or 0.05 mV in two contiguous leads in the absence of left ventricular hypertrophy or left bundle branch block is classified as a non-ST-segment elevation myocardial infarction (NSTEMI).

Courtesy of Thygesen, Alpert, & White, (2007).

---

**Digitalis and the EKG**

Digitalis can alter the EKG by causing (Adams-Hamoda, et al., 2003; Dubin, 2000; Garcia & Holtz, 2001):

- ST segment depression that is scooped or bowl-like (see Figure 9-18)
- Flat, depressed, or inverted T wave
- J point depression
- Shortened Q-T interval

**Figure 9-18   ST segment and digitalis**

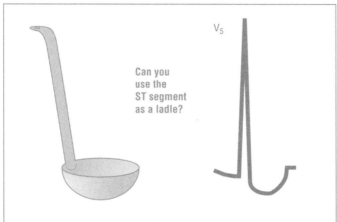

Can you
use the
ST segment
as a ladle?

$V_5$

*Source*: From *12-Lead ECG: The Art of Interpretation*, courtesy of Tomas B. Garcia, MD.

## T WAVE

The T-wave reflects ventricular repolarization (see Figure 9-19).

### Normal Conditions of the T Wave

- The T wave is present after each QRS complex.
- The T wave is "rounded and *asymmetric*" (Conover, 2003, p. 22).

**Figure 9-19 The T wave**

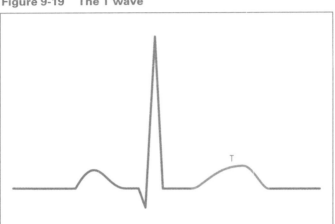

*Source*: From *12-Lead ECG: The Art of Interpretation*, courtesy of Tomas B. Garcia, MD.

- The T wave should be less than two-thirds the height of the R wave (Garcia & Holtz, 2001) or 5 mm (0.5 mV) or less in the limb leads, and 10 mm (1.0 mV) or less in the precordial leads (Adams-Hamoda, et al., 2003).
- The T wave is usually in the same direction as a narrow QRS complex except for leads $V_1$–$V_3$, where the T wave is opposite in deflection from the R wave. (Note: T waves may also be opposite in deflection from the R wave when the QRS is wide, e.g., bundle branch blocks.)
- The T wave is normally flipped or inverted in $aV_R$.

## Abnormal Conditions of the T Wave

- Symmetrical T waves may be seen with myocardial ischemia, central nervous system events, electrolyte abnormalities, and/or resolving pericarditis (Garcia & Holtz, 2001; see Figure 9-22).
- Tall, peaked, and narrow T waves may be seen with hyperkalemia, myocardial ischemia (Ganz, 2003), and/or short Q-T syndrome (Bjerregaard & Collier, 2004-2007).
- Broad T waves may be seen with long QT syndrome and central nervous system events, such as intracranial hemorrhage or stroke (Garcia & Holtz, 2001).
- Flipped or inverted may be seen with myocardial ischemia or myocardial injury (see Figure 9-23).

**Figure 9-22    A symmetrical T-wave can be a sign of pathology**

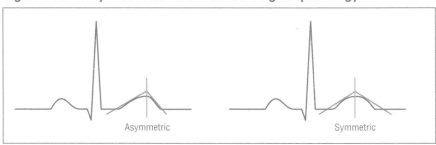

Asymmetric            Symmetric

*Source*: From *12-Lead ECG: The Art of Interpretation*, courtesy of Tomas B. Garcia, MD.

Other conditions associated with cause flipped or inverted T waves include (Adams-Hamoda, et al., 2003; Bresnahan & Eastwood, 2007; Ganz, 2003; Garcia & Holtz, 2001; Heiseman, 2007):

- Severe ventricular hypertrophy
- Pneumothorax
- Hypokalemia
- Pulmonary embolism (T wave inversion has an occurrence rate of 85%; Shaughnessy, 2007)
- Normal variant (4% of healthy patients can have a T wave inversion (Ganz, 2003)
- Left ventricular hypertrophy
- Digitalis
- Wellens syndrome causes marked T wave inversion in $V_2$ and $V_3$
  - Sign of critical stenosis in the left anterior descending coronary artery (Conover, 2003)

---

**T-wave Assessment Markers of a NSTEMI.**

- A T wave inversion with a depth greater than or equal to 1 mm (0.1 mV) in two contiguous leads with a prominent R wave or R:S ratio greater than 1 in the absence of left ventricular hypertrophy and left bundle branch block is classified as a non-ST-segment elevation myocardial infarction (NSTEMI) (ACC Clinical Data Standards, 2001; Thygesen, et al., 2007).

Note: The R:S ratio is the ratio of the amplitude of the R wave to the amplitude of the S wave (see Figure 9-23a).

---

**A Flipped or Inverted T Wave**

A flipped or inverted T wave (see Figure 9-23) in any lead except aVR, which is normally inverted, can occur within hours to days after an acute myocardial infarction (Achar, Kundu, & Norcross, 2005).

# U WAVE

It is controversial as to what causes the U wave (see Figure 9-24). Some postulate that it could be caused by ventricular repolarization of the Purkinje fibers, while others postulate that it could be caused by delayed mechanical relaxation of the ventricular myocardium (Ganz, 2003).

## Normal Conditions of the U Wave

- The U wave occurs between the T wave and the P wave, but it is often undetected because of its low voltage.
- The U wave is upright in all leads except $aV_R$, where it is inverted (Conover, 2003).
- The U wave can be seen best in chest leads $V_2$ and $V_3$ (Ganz, 2003), along with lead II (Sommargren & Drew, 2007).
- The U wave can be seen best in slower rhythms (Hebra, 1998).

**Figure 9-23a    Measuring the R:S ratio**

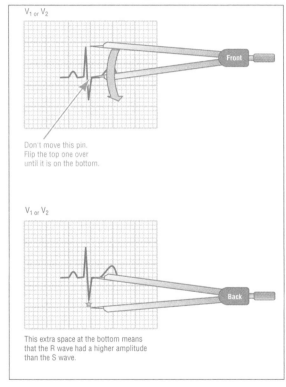

*Source*: From *12-Lead ECG: The Art of Interpretation*, courtesy of Tomas B. Garcia, MD.

**Figure 9-23   An inverted T wave**

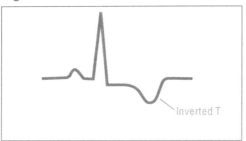

*Source*: Porter, W. *Porter's pocket guide to emergency and critical care*. Jones and Bartlett Publishers.

**Figure 9-24   The U wave**

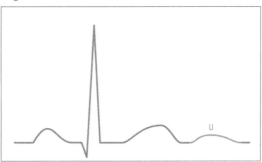

*Source*: From *12-Lead ECG: The Art of Interpretation*, courtesy of Tomas B. Garcia, MD.

**Figure 9-25   Extrapolate the T wave from the U wave**

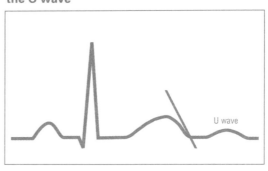

### The U Wave and the Q-T Interval

The U wave should be not be included in the measurement of the Q-T interval (ACC/AHA/HRS, 2006). To assist in extrapolating the T wave from the U wave, draw a diagonal line from the top of the T wave to the isoelectric line (see Figure 9-25).

## Abnormal Conditions of the U Wave

- A prominent U wave may be seen in hypokalemia, hypothermia, ischemia, postadministration of certain drugs, and long QT syndrome (Conover, 2003; Hebra, 1998; Ganz, 2003; Keller, 2008).
- "New onset U waves in normal sinus rhythm may be a precursor to the development of Torsades de Pointes" (Hebra, 1998, p. 31).
- An inverted U wave may be seen in heart disease and hypertension; the latter is the most common cause of an inverted U wave (Conover, 2003). An untreated U wave may also be seen with left anterior descording coronary artery ischemia.
- Prominent U waves may occur when there is a delay in ventricular repolarization (Devon, Ryan, Ochs, & Shapiro, 2008).

## Q-T INTERVAL

The Q-T interval (see Figure 9-26) reflects the interval of time from the beginning of ventricular depolarization to the end of ventricular repolarization. It is measured from the beginning of the QRS complex to the end of the T wave.

### Normal Conditions of the Q-T Interval

- The Q-T interval is normally less than or equal to 0.40 sec or 400 ms (American Heart Association, 2007f).
- The Q-T interval normally shortens with faster heart rates and lengthens with slower heart rates.
- Because the measured Q-T interval is affected by the patient's heart rate, it is important to calculate a QTc, particularly when the Q-T interval is lengthened or when the patient is on medications or has certain medical conditions that are known to prolong the interval.
- The QTc is a calculated number that corrects the QT interval for the patient's heart rate.
- The QTc is normally less than or equal to 0.44 or 440 ms in adult males and less than or equal to 0.46 or 460 ms in adult females (ACC/AHA/HRS, 2006).
- The Bazett formula is frequently used to calculate the QTc: QT divided by the square root of the preceding R-R interval (see Figures 9-27, 9-28, and 9-29).
  - Be sure to use the longest measured Q-T interval found on the rhythm strip.

**Figure 9-26   The QT interval**

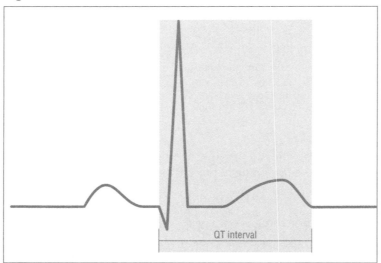

QT interval

*Source*: From *12-Lead ECG: The Art of Interpretation*, courtesy of Tomas B. Garcia, MD.

– To assist in finding the longest Q-T interval use the leads that have the most defined T waves. Rauen, Chulay, Bridges, Vollman, and Arbour (2008) suggest the use of lead II with continuous bedside EKG monitoring and the use of leads $V_3$ and $V_4$ with the 12-lead EKG.

– To calculate the QTc for patients in atrial fibrillation, identify the shortest R-R interval and the longest R-R interval. Calculate the QTc of each interval using the Bazett formula, then divide by two, as shown in the following equation (Al-Khatib, et al., 2003):

$$QTc = \frac{QTc \text{ (shortest R-R)} + QTc \text{ (longest R-R)}}{2}$$

– A limitation associated with the use of this formula is that is has been found to overestimate the QTc at high heart rates and underestimate the QTc at slow heart rates (Kupersmith, 1993).

**Figure 9-27    R-R interval**

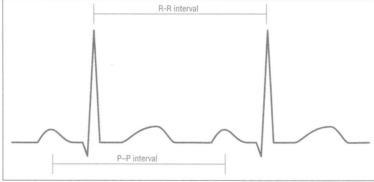

*Source*: From *12-Lead ECG: The Art of Interpretation*, courtesy of Tomas B. Garcia, MD.

**Figure 9-28    The authors QT (c) measurement**

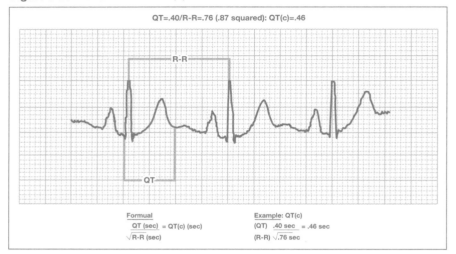

QT=.40/R-R=.76 (.87 squared): QT(c)=.46

Formual
$$\frac{QT\ (sec)}{\sqrt{R\text{-}R}\ (sec)} = QT(c)\ (sec)$$

Example: QT(c)
$$(QT)\ \frac{.40\ sec}{(R\text{-}R)\ \sqrt{.76}\ sec} = .46\ sec$$

**Figure 9-29    Square Root**

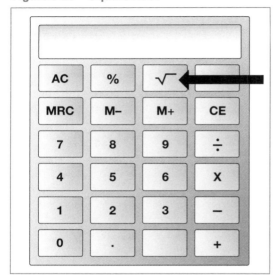

## Abnormal Conditions and Calculations of the of the Q-T Interval

Two abnormal conditions will be long Q-T and short Q-T

### Long QT

- A QTc greater than 0.44 sec or 440 ms for adult males and 0.46 sec or 460 ms for adult females is considered a long QT (ACC/AHA/HRS, 2006).

- A QTc greater than 0.50 sec or 500 ms is considered to be in the "danger zone" (Sommargren & Drew, 2007, p. 288). If left untreated, it can increase the risk of torsades de pointes and sudden death (torsades de pointes is a polymorphic (varying QRS shapes) ventricular tachycardia that can occur when there is prolongation of the Q-T interval).

• Overestimation of the QTc has also been found when bedside cardiac monitoring systems are used to calculate QTc (Rauen, et al., 2008) and when clinicians manually calculate the QTc (Taggart, Haglund, Tester, & Ackerman, 2007). When in doubt, use multiple leads or a 12-lead EKG rather than a single lead to identify the true QTc (Wagner & Lim, 2008a; Rauen, et al., 2008).

## CONGENITAL AND ACQUIRED CAUSE OF LONG QT

### Congenital Long QT Syndrome

• Congenital long QT syndrome (LQTS) is a genetic defect with an incidence of "1 in 3000" (Taggart, et al., 2007, p. 2620) that causes prolongation of the QTc interval in the absence of medications that prolong the interval.

  – Congenital long QT syndrome can often go unnoticed, so it is important to be attentive to unexplained signs and symptoms:

    ▪ Episodes of unexplained syncope or blackouts
    ▪ Family history of unexplained sudden cardiac death
    ▪ Family history of unexplained seizures

  – Genetic testing can be used to assist in identifying congenital LQTS. Two types of congenital LQTS are Romano-Ward syndrome and Jervell and Lange-Nielsen syndrome (Twedell, 2005).

---

**No Risk-Free Values for the QTc**

There are no QTc values that are considered to be free of risk (Al-Khatib, et al., 2003). Torsades de pointes can occur in patients with a QTc interval less than 0.50 sec (Rauen, et al., 2008), therefore, look for other warning signs that may occur prior to this arrhythmia, such as:

• Changes in the height and the polarity of the T wave (Keller, 2008.)
• Slower heart rates associated with pauses.
• New onset of a U wave (Hebra, 1998)

---

**Caution, Calculation, and QTc**

Use caution when calculating the QTc. One study found that 40% of patients had a QTc interval that was overestimated, which can lead to "inappropriate interventions and significant morbidity, both physical and emotional" (Taggart, et al., 2007, p. 2619–2620).

---

*Note:* Although lengthening of the Q-T interval can occur with subarachnoid hemorrhage, torsades de pointes rarely occurs in these patients (Sommargren & Drew, 2007).

## Acquired Long QT Syndrome

- Acquired Long QT syndrome is often associated with medications but various other conditions can prolong the Q-T interval such as:
    - Left ventricular wall hypertrophy (Sakata, et al., 2003).
    - Myocarditis (Keller, 2008).
    - Subarachnoid hemorrhage and acute cerebral trauma (Keller, 2008).
    - Electrolyte disorders, such as hypokalemia, hypocalcemia, and hypomagnesemia (Adams-Hamoda, et al., 2003; Al-Khatib, LaPointe, Kramer, & Califf, 2003; Keller, 2008; Sommargren & Drew, 2007).
    - Sudden drops in heart rate and compensatory pauses can predispose the patient to QT prolongation and can increase the risk of torsades de pointes.
    - Older age, female, starvation diets, ischemia, bradycardia, low ejection fractions, and metabolic conditions (Al-Khatib, et al., 2003; Sommargren & Drew, 2007).
    - The classification of medications that can prolong the QT interval include the following:
        - Antiarrhythmics
        - Antidepressant
        - Antipsychotic
        - Antibiotic
        - Antifungal
        - Antiviral

> *Note:* Amiodarone is an antiarrhythmic that is often used in the clinical setting to control rapid supraventricular arrhythmias and ventricular arrhythmias. Although amiodarone can prolong the Q-T interval by increasing repolarization time within the myocardial cell, there is a reduced risk of torsades de pointes because the drug "reduces transmural [all layers of the heart] dispersion" of ventricular repolarization (Keller, 2008, p. 79).

- ■ Anticancer
- ■ Antianginal
- ■ Antinausea
- – Careful monitoring of the Q-T interval should occur in the following circumstances:
  - ■ During initiation of medications that can prolong the Q-T interval
  - ■ Increase in the dosage of medications that can prolong the Q-T interval
  - ■ Overdosage of medications that can prolong the Q-T interval
- ■ Administration of multiple drugs known to prolong the Q-T interval, such as an antibiotic with an antiarrhythmic (Sommargren & Drew, 2007)

> *Note:* Women have a greater risk than men of developing drug-induced torsades de pointes (Keller, 2008).

> **QTc Measurements**
> QTc measurements should be performed at least every 8 hours on hospitalized patients who are on telemetry and are taking medications that can prolong the Q-T interval.

## Short Q-T

(Bjerregaard & Colleir, 2004-2007; U. S. National Library of Medicine, 2008b).

- A QTc less than 0.30 sec or 300 ms is considered a short QT (Reinig & Engel, 2007).
- Short QT syndrome (SQTS) is a rare congenital abnormality that is thought to alter the action potential and reduce repolarization time within the myocardial cells. The shortened refractory time increases the risk of abnormal arrhythmias such as atrial fibrillation and ventricular fibrillation. In SQTS these arrhythmias can occur without any structural heart disease (Poglagen, Fister, Radorancevic, & Vrtovec, 2006).
- Some patients do not have any signs and symptoms while others can have palpitations, unexplained syncopal episodes, dizziness, fainting, and sudden death.

# The Electrocardiogram

The electrocardiogram (EKG or ECG) provides the clinician with essential information to assist in determining the speed and the amount of electrical activity that is traveling through the different areas of the heart (American Heart Association, 2007c, Twedell, 2005). It also provides "information about the heart's resting and recovery phases" (Dubin, 1996, p. 7) and the directional flow of electrical activity:

- Speed of electrical activity
- Amount of electrical activity
- Rest and recovery phase of electrical activity
- Directional flow of electrical activity

EKG monitoring serves three primary purposes:

- To detect arrhythmias
- To detect myocardial ischemia, injury, and infarction
- To detect prolonged Q-T interval

**Additional Aspects of the Electrocardiogram**

- The EKG "remains a key tool in the diagnosis of Q-wave infarction" (Vacek, 2002, para. 2).
- The EKG can aid in identifying the culprit artery (s) in myocardial ischemia or myocardial infarction (Nair & Glancy, 2002).
- The EKG can provide the clinician with information that will assist in establishing a diagnosis, assist in stratifying the patient's risk of acute coronary syndrome, and assist in determining a treatment strategy (Achar, Kundu, & Norcross, 2005).
- "ECG remains one of the most important clinical tests in the evaluation of long QT syndrome" (Taggart, et al., 2007, p. 2614).
- "The EKG is the most common test used to diagnose arrhythmias" (National Heart Lung and Blood Institute, n.d., para. 5).
- The EKG provides the clinician with different views or snapshots of the electrical activity occurring throughout the heart, that is, an anterior view, lateral view, inferior view, and septal view (see Figure 10-1).

**Figure 10-1    The EKG takes snapshots of the heart**

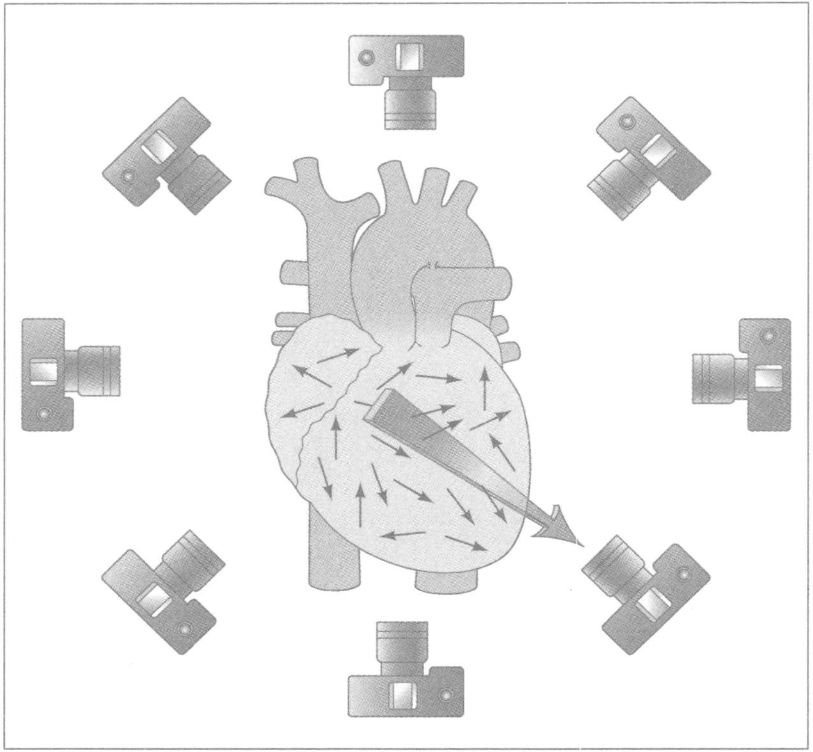

*Source*: From *12-Lead ECG: The Art of Interpretation*, courtesy of Tomas B. Garcia, MD.

## THE ELECTRICAL CURRENT/VECTOR

The direction of the electrical current or vector normally starts in the upper right aspect of the heart and travels down and to the left in a diagonal fashion. The reason that the vector travels down and to the left is because the greatest amount of muscle is in the left ventricle (see Figure 10-2).

This normal flow of electrical activity can be altered by:

> **Caution and the EKG**
>
> "A normal electrocardiogram does not rule out coronary syndrome" (Achar, et al., 2005, p. 120). In one study, 10% of patients who were admitted for chest pain had an acute coronary syndrome but presented with a normal EKG (Achar, et al., 2005).

- The position of the heart within the chest, that is, a horizontal position or a vertical position. Conditions that can alter the position of the heart within the chest include pneumothorax, obesity, older age, pregnancy (Adams-Hamoda, et al., 2003), and the height of the patient.
  - A horizontal position of the heart could shift the electrical current up and toward the left.
  - A vertical position of the heart could shift the electrical current down and toward the right.
- The condition of the electrical circuits within the heart, that is, electrical circuits that have been damaged by ischemia, injury, and/or infarction.
  - A lateral wall myocardial infarction or a right bundle branch block could shift the electrical current down and to the right.
  - An inferior myocardial infarction or a left bundle branch block could shift the electrical current up and toward the left.
- The structure of the heart, that is, hypertrophy.
  - Right ventricular hypertrophy could shift the electrical current down and toward the right.
  - Left ventricular hypertrophy could shift the electrical current up and toward the left.

## THE ELECTRICAL AXIS

The direction of depolarization that is spreading through the heart to stimulate a ventricular contraction determines the electrical axis (Dubin, 2000). Lead I and lead II are used to determine axis. Augmented unipolar leads, such as $aV_F$, are not recommended because the relative voltage and magnitude of the unipolar leads are not the same as the bipolar leads (American Heart Association, 2007b; see Figure 10-3).

A description of the axis deviations is as follows (American Heart Association, 2007b; Wagner & Lim, 2008a):

- Normal axis (flow is down and toward the left lower aspect of the heart between -30 to +90): Lead I = upright; lead II = upright
- Left axis deviation (flow is upward and to the left upper aspect of the heart -30 to -90): Lead I = upright; lead II = downward
- Right axis deviation (flow is downward and to the right +90 to +/-180): Lead I = downward; lead II = upright
- Extreme right axis deviation (flow is upward and to the right +/- 180 to -90): Lead I = downward; lead II = downward

## THE 3-LEAD, 5-LEAD, AND 12-LEAD EKG MONITORING SYSTEMS

Recording the electrical activity that is traveling through the heart can be accomplished through the three lead, five lead, or twelve lead systems.

**Figure 10-2   Normal direction of the electrical current/vector**

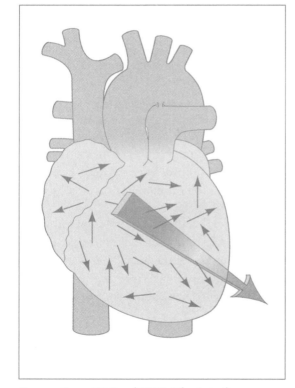

*Source*: From *12-Lead ECG: The Art of Interpretation*, courtesy of Tomas B. Garcia, MD.

**Figure 10-3    The electrical axis**

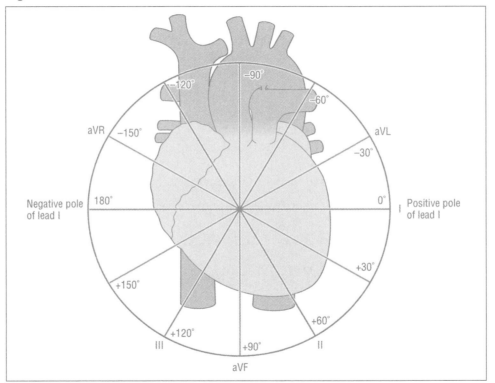

*Source*: From *12-Lead ECG: The Art of Interpretation*, courtesy of Tomas B. Garcia, MD.

## Three-Lead Systems and the Modified Leads

The three-lead systems provide limited views of the electrical activity of the heart.

- There are only three skin electrodes used in this system: a positive, a negative, and a ground.
- The leads that can be monitored with the three-lead systems are leads I, II, and III.
- A direct view of the V lead cannot be obtained unless the leads are repositioned on the patient's chest.
  - Leads that are repositioned on the patient's chest to obtain a view of the V lead are called modified leads.
  - Modified chest leads (MCL) *simulate* the V lead.
  - Modified chest leads should *not* be used when a direct view of the V lead can be obtained.

## Five-Lead Systems

The five-lead system is the most common method used for continuous cardiac monitoring.

- There are five skin electrodes used in this system: right arm, left arm, right leg, left leg, and the chest lead.
- A direct view of the V lead can be obtained.
- Leads that can be monitored with the five lead system are leads I, II, III, $aV_R$, $aV_L$, $aV_F$, and one chest lead.

### Placement of the Skin Electrodes and the Five-Lead System

- Right arm: Position under the right clavicle midclavicular line close to the junction of the right arm and torso.
- Left arm: Position under the left clavicle midclavicular line close to the junction of the left arm and torso.
- Right leg: Position at the level of the lowest rib midclavicular line on the right abdominal region. If necessary, the lead can also be placed on the right hip.

**Chest Lead Repositioning**

To monitor different chest leads, simply move the chest lead. Example: The clinician has been monitoring $V_1$ but would like to begin to monitor $V_6$. To obtain a view of $V_6$, move the chest lead from $V_1$ (fourth intercostal space to the right of the sternum) to $V_6$ (horizontal plane of $V_4$ to the left of the sternum midaxillary line).

- Left leg: Position at the level of the lowest rib midclavicular line on the left abdominal region. If necessary, the lead can also be placed on the left hip.
- Chest (Precordial) lead: Position at the site that will display the V lead that is selected to be monitored (see "Placement of the Six Precordial Lead Electrodes and the Standard 12-lead EKG" later in this section).

## 12-Lead Systems

The standard 12-lead system (see Figure 10-4) takes a 10-sec snapshot of the electrical activity of the heart from 12 different angles.

- The 12-lead system uses 10 skin electrodes to obtain 12 pictures of the heart. There are four limb lead electrodes and six precordial lead electrodes.
- A direct view of all chest leads can be obtained at the same time.
- Leads that can be monitored with the 12-lead systems are: I, II, III, $aV_R$, $aV_L$, $aV_F$, $V_1$, $V_2$, $V_3$, $V_4$, $V_5$, and $V_6$.
- While a standard 12-lead system can provide the clinician with a great amount of information, it can miss ischemic events and arrhythmias because it only records 10 sec of electrical activity.

### Placement of the Four Limb Lead Electrodes for the Standard 12-Lead EKG

The Society for Cardiological Science & Technology (2006) recommends placing the four limb lead electrodes for the standard 12-lead EKG as follows:

- Right arm limb lead (RA, red): Right forearm, proximal to the wrist
- Left arm limb lead (LA, yellow): Left forearm, proximal to the wrist
- Left leg limb lead (LL, green): Left lower leg, proximal to the ankle
- Right leg limb lead (RL, black): Right lower leg, proximal to the ankle

*Note:* The limb leads should be positioned on the distal limbs. If it is necessary to move the limb leads from the distal limbs to the torso, it is important to make a notation on the EKG because this change can alter the appearance of the EKG (The Society for Cardiological Science & Technology, 2006).

## Placement of the Six Precordial Lead Electrodes for the Standard 12-Lead EKG

- $V_1$: Fourth intercostal space to the right of the sternum
- $V_2$: Fourth intercostal space to the left of the sternum
- $V_3$: Positioned between $V_2$ and $V_4$
- $V_4$: Fifth intercostal space to the left of the sternum midclavicular line
- $V_5$: Horizontal plane of $V_4$ to the left of the sternum anterior axillary line (if the anterior axillary line is hard to find, place $V_5$ between $V_4$ and $V_6$)
- $V_6$: Horizontal plane of $V_4$ to left of the sternum midaxillary line

## Two Ways to Properly Position the Precordial Leads Electrodes

When positioning the precordial leads on the patient's chest, it is important to manually palpate the intercostal spaces. There are two ways this can be accomplished:

- The first approach uses the clavicle.
  1. Find the clavicle (the clavicle sits on top of the first rib).
  2. After the clavicle has been identified, let your fingers slide down to locate the first intercostal space, but avoid counting the small space that exists between the clavicle and the first rib (The Society for Cardiological Science & Technology, 2006).

**Figure 10-4   The 12 leads of the ECG**

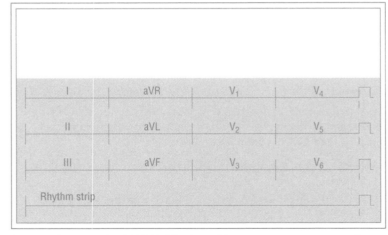

*Source*: From *12-Lead ECG: The Art of Interpretation*, courtesy of Tomas B. Garcia, MD.

3. Using the ribs as landmarks, palpate down three more spaces from the first intercostal space to find the fourth intercostal space.

4. $V_1$ sits at the fourth intercostal space to the right of the sternum.

- The second approach uses the manubrium (the broad upper part of the sternum).

    1. Find the bump where the manubrium joins the sternum (this is known as the Louis angle). The Louis angle is at the level of the second intercostal space.

    2. Palpate down two spaces from the Louis angle to find the fourth intercostal space.

    3. $V_1$ sits at the fourth intercostal space to the right of the sternum.

## Other Things to Consider When Positioning the Precordial Leads

Figure 10-5 demonstrates the lead placement for the 12-lead EKG.

- Place all precordial leads under the breast (Kligfield, et al., 2007a).

- Misplacement of the precordial leads can result in erroneous assessments. Common errors that have been found include:

    – Placement of the lateral precordial leads too low (The Society for Cardiological Science & Technology, 2006).

    – Placement of $V_1$ and $V_2$ too high (the incorrect placement of $V_1$ and $V_2$ can look like poor R wave progression and anterior infarction on the EKG, and this can lead to a misdiagnosis (Kligfield, Mason, & Gettes, 2007b)

**R Wave Progression**

A normal R wave progression (see Figure 10-6) results when electrical activity traveling across the precordial leads from $V_1$ to $V_4$–$V_5$, causes the R wave to increase in amplitude and exceed the S wave in a consecutive fashion (Ganz, 2003). An anterior myocardial infarction is one condition that can cause poor R wave progression.

**Figure 10-5    Lead placement for the 12-lead EKG**

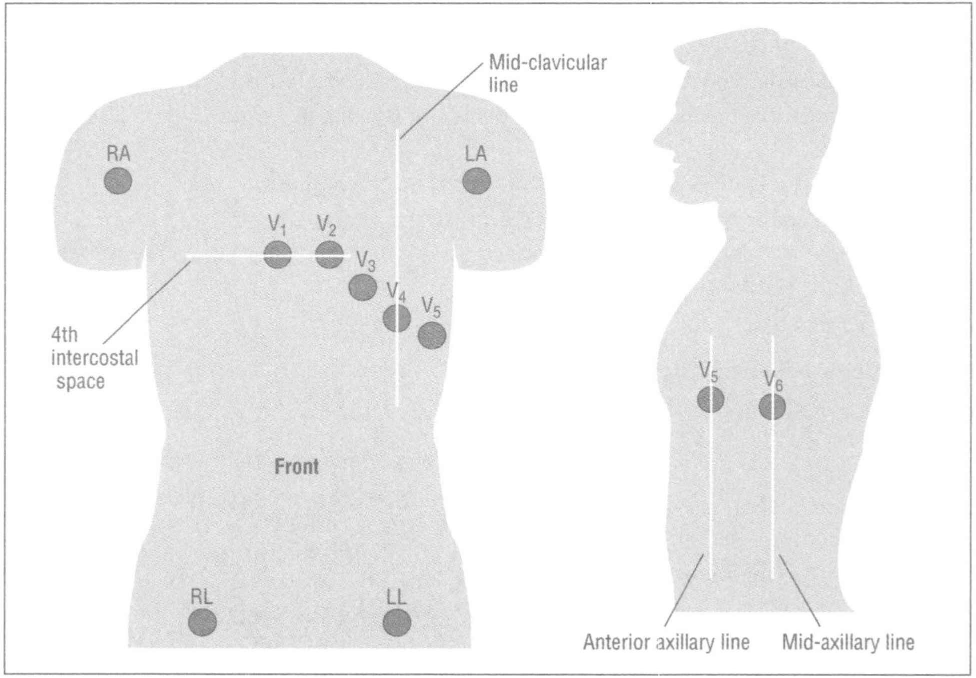

*Source*: From *12-Lead ECG: The Art of Interpretation*, courtesy of Tomas B. Garcia, MD.

**Figure 10-6    R-wave progression**

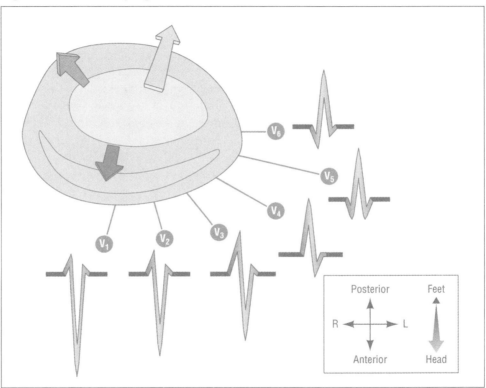

*Source*: From *12-Lead ECG: The Art of Interpretation*, courtesy of Tomas B. Garcia, MD.

## DERIVED 12-LEAD MONITORING SYSTEMS

The use of 10 skin electrodes to obtain a continuous 12-lead EKG monitoring is challenging in the clinical setting. To address this issue, the EASI system was developed in 1980 by Dower and colleagues.

- The EASI system is a 12-lead EKG system that uses only five skin electrodes along with mathematical calculations to create a **derived** 12-lead EKG.
- Because this system is continuous, it can assist in improving assessments and interpretations of EKG rhythms and ST segment ischemic episodes that could be missed with the standard 12-lead snapshot (Jahrsdoerfer, Guiliano& Stephens, 2005).
- Although continuous-derived 12-lead monitoring systems can be useful in the clinical setting (Booker, et al., 2003; Drew, 2002; Flanders, 2007), there are some drawbacks:
  - They should not be used to compare serial EKGs.
  - "They cannot be considered equivalent to standard 12-lead recordings or recommended at present as an alternative for routine use" (Kligfield, et al., 2007a, p. 1120).

The placement of the five skin electrodes with the EASI system is as follows:

- Lower part of the sternum (E)
- Left midaxilla fifth intercostal space (A)
- Upper part of the sternum (manubrium) (S)
- Right midaxilla fifth intercostal space (I)
- Anywhere that is convenient on the torso (reference electrode)

# The EKG Leads and Electrical Activity

## NEGATIVE AND POSITIVE ELECTRODES

The skin electrodes that are placed on the patient limbs and precordium are assigned a specific polarity, either a positive polarity or a negative polarity. The measured difference in voltage potential between the selected polarized electrodes produces the EKG tracings.

> *Note:* The polarity of the electrode is dependent on what lead is being viewed. For example, in Lead I the left arm (LA) skin electrode is positive but in Lead III the left arm (LA) skin electrode is negative.

- All electrical activity is recorded at the positive electrode.
- If the electrical activity (wave of depolarization) is moving toward the positive electrode, there will be an upward deflection of the EKG complex.
- If the electrical activity (wave of depolarization) is moving away from the positive electrode, there will be a downward deflection of the EKG complex.
- If the electrical activity (wave of depolarization) is moving partially toward and partially away from the positive electrode there will be an upward and a downward deflection of the EKG complex (see Figure 11-1).

## THE 12 LEADS AND ELECTRICAL ACTIVITY

Please see Figure 11-2 for a diagram of the 12 leads and electrical activity.

The standard 12-lead EKG consists of six limb leads (three standard limb leads and three augmented limb leads) and six chest (precordial) leads.

**Figure 11-1 Electrical activity and the deflection of the QRS**

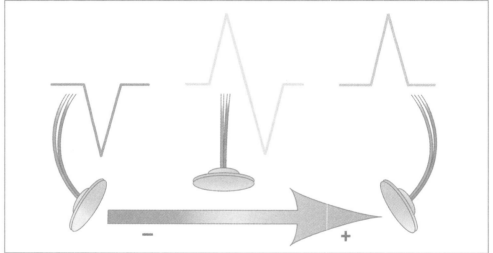

*Source*: From *12-Lead ECG: The Art of Interpretation*, courtesy of Tomas B. Garcia, MD.

- Leads I, II, and III (the standard limb leads) are bipolar leads, that is, they measure the difference in voltage potential between two electrodes: a negatively polarized electrode and a positively polarized electrode.

- Leads $aV_R$, $aV_L$, $aV_F$, (the augmented leads) and $V_1$–$V_6$ (the chest leads) are unipolar leads, that is, they measure the difference in voltage potential at the specific location of the heart where the skin electrode is placed using one electrode: a positively polarized electrode.

> *Note:* The unipolar leads use the center of the heart as the null or zero reference point.

> *Note:* The limb leads record electrical activity in the frontal plane.

## Six Limb Leads (I, II, III, $aV_R$, $aV_L$, $aV_F$)

- Lead I: Measures the electrical difference between the negative electrode on the right arm and the positive electrode on the left arm across the base of the heart.
  - The R wave is upright.
  - Lead I can be useful in viewing the electrical activity in the high lateral wall of the left ventricle.

**Augmented Leads**
Augmented means there is an increase in the voltage and magnitude of the electrical activity that is being recorded.

- Lead II: Measures the electrical difference between the negative electrode on the right arm and the positive electrode on the left leg.
  - The R wave is upright.
  - Lead II can be useful in viewing the electrical activity in the inferior wall of the heart.
- Lead III: Measures the electrical difference between the negative electrode on the left arm and the positive electrode on the left leg.
  - The R wave is upright.
  - Lead III can be useful in viewing the electrical activity in the inferior wall of the heart.

**Figure 11-2   The 12 leads and the EKG**

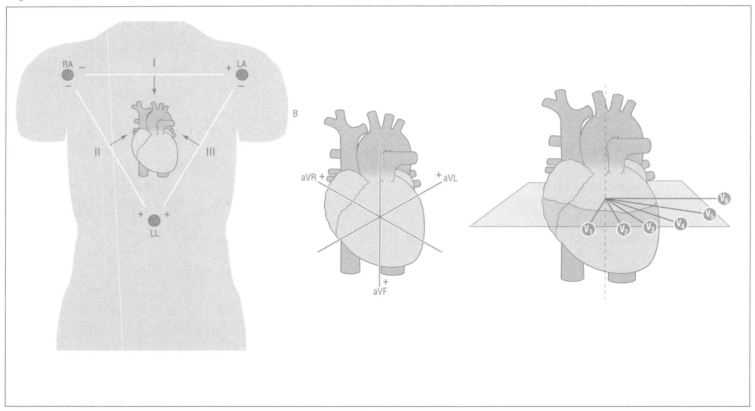

- $aV_R$ (augmented voltage of right arm): Measures the electrical activity of the electrode on the right arm.
  - The R wave is downward.
  - $aV_R$ should have flipped T waves and flipped U waves.
  - $aV_R$ is often ignored in ECG analysis, however, here are a few examples of the clinical usefulness of this lead:
    - ST segment elevation in $aV_R$ during exercise testing has been shown to be associated with left anterior descending (LAD) coronary artery stenosis (Neill, et al., 2007).
    - "Yamaji and associates (as cited in Nair & Glancy, 2002) found ST-segment elevation to occur more frequently in lead $aV_R$ than in any other lead in patients with acute left main coronary arterial obstruction" (p. 138).
    - Nair & Glancy, 2002, report that S-T segment depression in $aV_R$ may be useful in distinguishing a right coronary artery occlusion from a left circumflex artery occlusion in an acute inferior myocardial infarction.
- $aV_L$ (augmented voltage of left arm): Measures the electrical activity of the electrode on the left arm.
  - The R wave is usually upward.
  - $aV_L$ can be useful in viewing electrical activity in the high lateral wall of the left ventricle.
- $aV_F$ (augmented voltage of left foot): Measures the electrical activity of the electrode on the left foot.
  - The R wave is upward.
  - $aV_F$ can be useful in viewing the electrical activity in the inferior wall of the heart.

## Six Chest (Precordial) Leads ($V_1$–$V_6$)

- $V_1$: Measures the electrical activity at the fourth inter-costal space to the right of the sternum.
  - The R wave is predominantly downward.
  - $V_1$ is helpful in differentiating supraventricular arrhythmias from ventricular arrhythmias.

> Note: The precordial leads record the electrical activity of the left ventricle in the horizontal plane.

- $V_1$ can assist in identifying atrial enlargement, ventricular hypertrophy, and the type of bundle branch block.

- $V_2$: Measures the electrical activity at the fourth intercostal space to the left of the sternum.
  - The R wave is predominantly downward.
  - $V_2$ can be useful in viewing electrical activity in the interventricular septum and the anterior wall of the left ventricle.

- $V_3$: Measures the electrical activity occurring between the $V_2$ and $V_4$ leads (this lead is positioned between $V_2$ and $V_4$).
  - The R wave is equiphasic (it has a mixture of upward and downward waveforms).
  - $V_3$ can be useful in viewing electrical activity in the interventricular septum and the anterior wall of the left ventricle.

- $V_4$: Measures the electrical activity at the fifth intercostal space to the left of the sternum at the midclavicular line.
  - The R wave is predominantly upward.
  - $V_4$ can be useful in viewing electrical activity of the anterior wall of the left ventricle.

- $V_5$: Measures the electrical activity along the horizontal plane of $V_4$ to the left of the sternum at the anterior axillary line.
  - The R wave is upward.
  - $V_5$ can be useful in viewing the electrical activity of the low lateral wall of the left ventricle.

- $V_6$: Measures the electrical activity along the horizontal plane of $V_4$ to the left of the sternum at the midaxillary line (Kligfield, et al., 2007a).
  - The R wave is upward and is often a mirror image of $V_1$ when inverted.
  - $V_6$ can be useful in viewing the electrical activity of the low lateral wall of the left ventricle.

> *Note:* If the anterior axillary line is difficult to find, place the $V_5$ electrode midway between $V_4$ and $V_6$ (Kligfield, et al., 2007a).

## RIGHT CHEST LEADS (V$_1$R-V$_6$R)

A right-side 12-lead EKG should be obtained to record the electrical activity of the right ventricle if the clinician suspects any of the following:

- Right ventricular hypertrophy
- Right ventricular infarction (common after an acute inferior wall myocardial infarction)
- Dextrocardia (displacement of the heart to the right side of the chest)

A right-side EKG is obtained by placing the precordial leads to the right of the sternum.

- V$_1$R: Position to the left of the sternum fourth intercostal space
- V$_2$R: Position to the right of the sternum fourth intercostal space
- V$_3$R: Position halfway between V$_2$R and V$_4$R
- V$_4$R: Position to the right of the sternum fifth intercostal space, right midclavicular line
- V$_5$R: Position to the right of the sternum along the horizontal plane of V$_4$R at the anterior axillary line
- V$_6$R: Position to the right of the sternum along the horizontal plane of V$_4$R at the midaxillary line
- The limb leads are not repositioned

**Acute Inferior Myocardial Infarctions and Right Ventricular Infarction**

- Right ventricular infarction occurs in one-third to one-half of patients with an acute inferior myocardial infarction (Carter & Ellis, 2005; Levin, 2008).
- It is highly suggested, therefore, to routinely perform a right-side 12-lead EKG when a patient presents with an acute inferior myocardial infarction.
- Time is of the essence because the ST segment elevation can resolve within 10–12 hr from the onset of signs and symptoms (Carter & Ellis, 2005).

**Right Ventricular Infarction**

ST segment elevation in leads V$_3$R and V$_4$R is highly suggestive of a right ventricular infarction (Carter & Ellis, 2005; Thygesen, et al., 2007).

## LEAD SELECTION FOR CONTINUOUS EKG MONITORING

Lead selection is dependent on the patient's history, the reason for admission, and the reason for continuously monitoring electrical signals that are traveling through the patient's heart. To assist in choosing the best lead for continuous EKG monitoring, the clinician can ask the following questions:

- Why does the patient require continuous monitoring?
- What lead will offer the most information based on the patient's condition?
- What should I anticipate to see during continuous monitoring of the patient?

**Dextrocardia and Swapping the Limb Leads**
- An inverted P-wave on lead I of a right-side 12-lead EKG can serve as a diagnostic clue for dextrocardia.
- "Swapping of the right and left limb leads", when performing a right-side 12-lead EKG, "will 'normalize' the appearance of the limb leads," and the inverted P wave will not be seen.
- If the clinician prefers to swap the limb leads be sure to clearly document this on the EKG so dextrocardia is not overlooked (The Society for Cardiological Science & Technology, 2006, p. 10).

When choosing a lead(s) for continuous EKG monitoring, be sure to use the lead(s) that provide the best picture of what needs to be monitored:

- Detection of arrhythmias
- Detection of ischemia
- Detection of prolongation of the Q-T interval

### Suggested Leads for the Detection of Arrhythmias (II, $V_1$, $V_6$)

- Leads $V_1$ or $V_6$ are suggested for ventricular arrhythmias to assist in differentiation between aberrancy versus ectopy.
- Leads II, III, or VF are suggested for atrial arrhythmias to assist in identifying atrial fibrillation versus atrial flutter.

*Note:* Ischemia can occur in patients who have chest pain without ST segment changes and in patients who have ST segment changes without chest pain (Alpert, et al., 2000).

- Lead $V_1$ can provide a good view of the P waves and the QRS morphology and, therefore, is a suggested lead to use to differentiate supraventricular tachycardia (SVT) from ventricular tachycardia (VT) (Drew, 2002).
- $V_1$ is preferred over MCL[1] because $V_1$ provides a direct view of the electrical morphology of the heart (Drew, 2002).

## Suggested Leads for Detection of Ischemia Using the ST Segment (III & $V_3$; with a stable coronary artery III & $V_5$)

- Selecting a lead that will identify ischemia is important because 80–90% of ischemic events are clinically silent (Drew, 2002; Drew & Krucoff, 1999; Flanders, 2007).
- Failure to identify ischemia can lead to poorer patient outcomes (Devon, et al., 2008; Pelter, Adams, & Drew, 2002).
- Suggested leads to use for ST segment monitoring specific for the coronary artery includes:
  - Right coronary artery (RCA): III, $aV_F$
  - Left anterior descending (LAD) coronary artery: $V_2$, $V_3$, $V_4$
  - Left circumflex coronary artery: $V_3$ (often electrically "silent" on EKG)
  - Unknown coronary artery: III, $V_3$
  - Stable coronary artery: $V_5$ can be used to pick up ischemic events during exercise and/or ambulation (Drew & Krucoff, 1999)
  - To optimize the ability to identify ischemic events, monitor as many leads as possible (Flanders, 2007).
- For ST segment monitoring to be effective, it is important that a baseline ST segment be identified for each individual patient because conditions such as ventricular hypertrophy, digitalis therapy, and conduction abnormalities can alter the patient's ST segment. If a baseline is not established, ischemic events can be misinterpreted. For example, a patient with ventricular hypertrophy has an ST segment that is normally depressed by 1 mm. When the patient becomes ischemic, the ST segment rises up to the isoelectric line and appears to be normal (this is called pseudonormalization). If the baseline ST segment was not established, this ischemic event could be missed.

## Suggested Leads for Detection of Prolongation of the QT ($V_3$, $V_4$, II)

- Although precordial leads $V_1$–$V_6$ can be used to measure the Q-T interval because they reflect "local ventricular activity" (Sakata, et al., 2003, p. 885), $V_3$ and $V_4$ are the most reliable leads for QT measurements (Keller, 2008).
- Lead II can assist in identification of the U wave (Sommargren & Drew, 2007), which is helpful because the U wave should not be included in the calculation of the Q-T interval.

**Table 11-1   Summary of Suggested EKG Leads**

| | |
|---|---|
| Arrhythmias | Suggested leads II, $V_1$, $V_6$ |
| Ischemia = ST segment monitoring | Suggested leads III, $V_3$; if stable coronary artery use III, $V_5$ |
| Prolongation of the QT | Suggested leads $V_3$, $V_4$, II |

# SECTION 12

# The Best Picture

Obtaining the best picture of the electrical activity traveling through the heart can provide the clinician with information that will assist to analyze, diagnose, and treat the patient in a timely manner. The following strategies can used to obtain the "Best Picture":

- Prepare the skin.
- Attach the EKG electrodes/tabs
- Monitor the graph paper
- Minimize artifact

## PREPARE THE SKIN

- Clear the chest of excess body hair by shaving the patient if needed. Be sure to obtain verbal consent from the patient if shaving is necessary (The Society for Cardiological Science & Technology, 2006).

> *Note:* If there is a chance that the patient may need surgery, use an electric razor to clip the patient's chest hair (Nichols, 2001).

- Cleanse the skin at all electrode sites with mild soap, alcohol, or skin prep pads to remove surface oils from the skin. Be careful with patients who have sensitive or broken skin (The Society for Cardiological Science & Technology, 2006).
- Rub the skin dry at all electrode sites with a gauze swab, paper towel, or abrasive tape to exfoliate the skin. Cleaning and gentle abrasion can reduce artifact (Kligfield, et al., 2007a).
- If the patient is diaphoretic, consider the use of a tincture of benzoin if the patient has no known allergy to it. Specifically formulated skin preparation gels and pads can also be used to increase adhesion to the skin.

## ATTACH THE EKG ELECTRODES/TABS

- Stress test vests and/or sweaters can be used to hold patient lead wires and electrodes in place during continuous 12-lead EKG monitoring, Holter monitoring, or during stress tests.
- Check the center of the electrode to ensure it is moist, and do not contaminate this moist area with gels, powders, or lotions.
- Attach electrodes to the lead wire prior to placement on the chest.
- Correctly identify the location of the leads to ensure proper placement on the patient's skin. Incorrect lead placement can alter the morphology of the EKG complexes (Castellanos, Pastor, Zambrano, & Myerburg, 2002; Kligfield, et al., 2007a).
- Mark the electrode sites with indelible ink so the electrodes remain in the same location when replaced (Conover, 2003).
- Move the electrodes if the skin becomes irritated.
- Hypoallergenic electrodes can be used if necessary.
- When replacement of one electrode is needed, replace all of the electrodes.
- All electrodes should be the same brand.
- If the patient is on telemetry, be sure to replace the batteries often to ensure proper amplitude of the EKG complexes.
- Do not place electrodes over a pacemaker.
- If the lead wires become dark in appearance, frayed, stiff, or cut, they should be replaced.

## MONITOR THE GRAPH PAPER

- Speed of the graph paper:
  - The sweep speed of the graph paper used for continuous cardiac monitoring is normally 25 mm/sec (Homoud, 2008).
  - If a clinician is having difficulty with identification of the electrical activity of the heart, the sweep speed can be increased from 25 mm/sec to 50 mm/sec (Sommargren & Drew, 2007). This makes the EKG complex easier to read but it can cause the following:
    - Distortion of the complex because the complex widens out.

- ■ Difficulty when comparing this EKG with an EKG at 25 mm/sec
- Calibration box on the graph paper (see Figure 12-1):
  - – Standard calibration: 10 mm or 1 mV high, 0.20 sec wide (Figure 12-1, A).
  - – Half-standard calibration (stairlike): Seen when the complexes are so tall that they run into each other (Figure 12-1, B).
  - – Large calibration: Seen when the paper speed is increased from 25 mm/sec to 50 mm/sec. If the speed is increased to 50 mm, the calibration box will be 10 mm high and 0.40 sec wide (Garcia & Holtz, 2001) (Figure 12-1, C).

## MINIMIZE ARTIFACT

- Artifact can trigger alarms and can interfere with analysis of the EKG. Any time an alarm is triggered, assess the patient to determine if the alarm was triggered by an arrhythmia or by artifact. Two examples of activities that can produce artifact include:
  - – Respiratory vest therapy, used to ensure effective airway clearance, can cause artifact that looks like ventricular tachycardia (Adams & Pelter, 2005).
  - – Body movements associated with activities such as brushing of teeth can cause artifact that looks like ventricular tachycardia (Mascitelli & Pezzetta, 2006).
- Artifact can be reduced when performing a 12-lead EKG by ensuring that the patient is as comfortable as possible and the limbs are still and relaxed.
- Artifact can be reduced by turning the filter on if necessary when performing a 12-lead EKG. The current recommendation, however, is to only use the filter when all attempts to eliminate interference have failed (The Society for Cardiological Science & Technology, 2006).

**Figure 12-1    Calibration boxes**

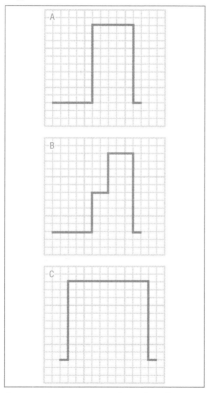

*Source*: From *12-Lead ECG: The Art of Interpretation*, courtesy of Tomas B. Garcia, MD.

- Artifact can be reduced by following the recommended recording bandwidth recommendations when performing a 12-lead EKG:
  - The low frequency cutoff should be no higher than "0.05 Hz for routine filters" to avoid distortion of the ST segment. This requirement can be relaxed to "0.67 Hz for linear digital filters with zero phase distortion" (Kligfield, et al., 2007a, p. 1112).
  - The high frequency cutoff for digital filters should be 150 Hz for adults, adolescents, and children and 250 Hz for infants "to reduce amplitude error measurements" (Kligfield, et al., 2007a, p. 1113).
- Artifact and erroneous readings can be reduced by ensuring that the electrodes are correctly placed on the patient, that is, the left arm on the left arm and not the left leg. Reversing the position of the leads can distort the EKG recording (Kligfield, et al., 2007a, p. 1121).

# SECTION 13

# Measurements, Calculations, and Documentation

## MILLIMETERS, MILLIVOLTS, AND DURATION OF TIME IN SECONDS

- The seconds or duration of time of the ECG complex is measured horizontally on the EKG graph paper (see Figure 13-1):
  - Each 1 mm box on the x axis (horizontal) = 0.04 sec
  - Five 1 mm boxes (5 mm) = 0.20 sec
  - Thirty 5 mm boxes = 6 sec
- The millivolts or amplitude of the ECG complex is measured vertically on the EKG graph paper(see Figure 13-1):
  - Each 1 mm box on the y axis (vertical) = 0.1 mV
  - Five 1 mm boxes (5 mm) = 0.5 mV
  - Ten 1 mm boxes (10 mm) = 1mV

## USE OF CALIPERS FOR MANUAL MEASUREMENTS

Utilize a caliper when performing manual measurements of rhythm strips. To assist in obtaining accurate measurements when using a caliper:

- Be sure the caliper has an adequate amount of tension.
- Move the caliper to a clean area on the graph paper and position it at the beginning of a 0.20 sec box (see Figure 13-2).

**Figure 13-1    Where to find seconds and millivolts on the ECG paper**

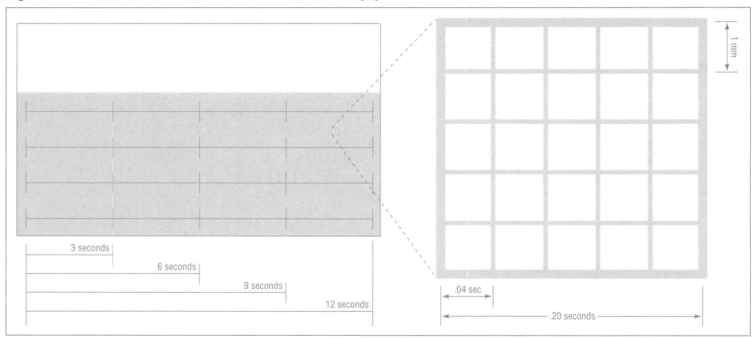

*Source*: From *12-Lead ECG: The Art of Interpretation*, courtesy of Tomas B. Garcia, MD.

## COMPUTER-BASED ANALYSIS VERSUS MANUAL ANALYSIS OF THE EKG

- Errors have been found when alarms are triggered by automatic computerized measurements of ST segments, therefore a manual check of ST segments is always warranted (Eskola, et al., 2005).
- Overestimation of QTc has also been found when bedside cardiac monitoring systems are used to calculate QTc (Rauen, et al., 2008) and when clinicians manually calculate the QTc (Taggart, et al., 2007). When in doubt, use multiple leads or a 12-lead EKG rather than a single lead to identify the true QTc (Wagner & Lim, 2008a; Rauen, et al., 2008).
- "All computer-based reports require physician overreading" because it has been shown that physician analysis is more accurate than computer analysis (Kligfield, et al., 2007a, p. 1122).

## CALCULATION OF THE HEART RATE

The following strategies can be used to assist in calculating the heart rate from the EKG graph paper:

- (300, 150, 100) (75, 60, 50), (43, 38, 33) (Dubin, 2000; see Figures 13-3 and 13-4).

Memorizing these number groupings can assist the clinician to quickly determine the heart rate range.

**Figure 13-2   How to use the calipers effectively**

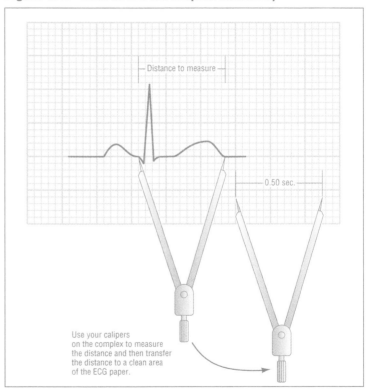

Distance to measure

0.50 sec.

Use your calipers on the complex to measure the distance and then transfer the distance to a clean area of the ECG paper.

*Source*: From *12-Lead ECG: The Art of Interpretation*, courtesy of Tomas B. Garcia, MD.

**Figure 13-3   Calculating the heart rate**

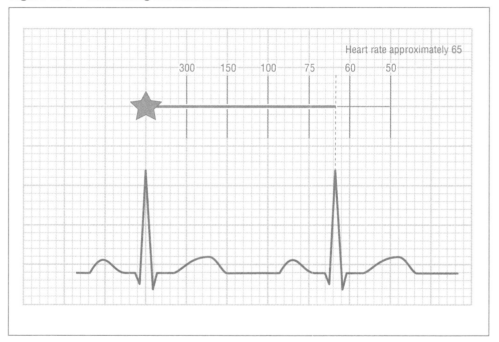

*Source*: From *12-Lead ECG: The Art of Interpretation*, courtesy of Tomas B. Garcia, MD.

**Figure 13-4    Tip: Use the thick lines found on the x axis (horizontal).**

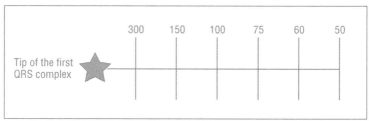

*Source*: From *12-Lead ECG: The Art of Interpretation*, courtesy of Tomas B. Garcia, MD.

- Count the R waves in a 6-sec strip and multiply by 10. Identify a 6-sec strip by:
  - Locating the small vertical or horizontal lines (hash marks) at the top of the paper. Three consecutive lines = 6 sec.
  - Counting out thirty 5 mm boxes on the graph paper (0.20 sec squares × 30 = 6 sec).

**PVCs and Heart Rate**

Isolated premature ventricular contractions (PVCs) that cause contractility of the heart should be counted into the calculation of the heart rate.

## DOCUMENTATION

- Use at least a 6 sec rhythm strip for analysis and for documentation. Be sure to include a readable strip that does not need to be folded over onto itself. If the strip is long, cut it into two pieces, and then place each piece consecutively in the chart.
- If the lead that is documented in the chart has been changed, note this change on the EKG strip. Example: *Lead has been changed from II to III.*
- If the position of the EKG patches on the patient's chest have been changed, note this change on the EKG. Example: *The V lead has been changed from a $V_1$ position to a $V_3$ position.*
- Document any rhythm change before and after treatment.
- Document any ischemic change before and after treatment.
- Document any prolongation of the Q-T interval before and after modifications in treatment.
- Document any dressings that interfere with proper EKG lead placement.
- Document anything that could cause a misreading or misinterpretation of the EKG. Examples: *Patient has sequential compression devices (SCDs). Patient is being externally paced.*
- Document if the chest leads were moved to the right side of the chest to obtain a right-side 12-lead EKG. Be sure to also document if the position of the limb leads was changed.
- Document if the 12-lead is from a derived system. Example: *EASI system being used for continuous monitoring.*
- Document any change in the patient's body position when a 12-lead EKG is recorded because the current recommendation is to record a 12-lead in the supine position (Kligfield, et al., 2007a). Examples: *Patient lying on left side. Patient lying on right side. Patient in prone position. Patient walking the halls. Patient sitting in wheelchair.*

# SECTION 14

# Eight-Step Method for Rhythm Strip Analysis

1. Rate
   - a. Normal (60–100 beats per min)
   - b. Bradycardia (< 60 beats per min)
   - c. Tachycardia (> 100 beats per min)
2. Rhythm
   - a. Regular
   - b. Irregular
3. P waves
   - a. P wave occurs before each QRS complex
   - b. P waves look the same in shape and in size
   - c. P waves in $V_1$ are monophasic, < 0.12 sec in duration, < 2.5 mm (0.25 mV) in height
   - d. P waves cannot be found
4. P-R interval
   - a. Normal (0.12 sec to 0.20 sec)
   - b. Short (< 0.12 sec)
   - c. Long (> 0.20 sec)
   - d. Cannot determine

5. QRS complex
   a. QRS complex occurs after each P wave
   b. QRS complexes look the same in shape and size
   c. QRS complex is normal (< 0.12 sec)
   d. QRS complex is wide (≥ 0.12 sec)
6. QRS complex direction in $V_1$
   a. Negative
   b. Positive
   c. Cannot determine
7. Q-T interval
   a. Normal (≤ 0.40 sec)
8. QTc
   a. Normal (men ≤ 0.44 sec, women ≤ 0.46 sec)
   b. Long or approaching the danger zone (> 0.50 sec)

# Speedy Six-Step Method for 12-Lead EKG Analysis

## SPEEDY SIX-STEP METHOD

1. Check the calibration box and the sweep speed.
   a. The standard calibration box, which can be found on the EKG, is 10 mm or 1 mV high and 0.20 sec wide (Garcia & Holtz, 2001), and the sweep speed of the graph paper is normally 25 mm/sec (Homoud, 2008).
2. Use the long continuous rhythm strip, if available, on the 12-lead EKG, and perform the eight-step method for rhythm strip analysis (see Figure 15-1 and Section 14).
3. Determine the electrical axis (see Figure 15-2 and Table 15-1).
4. Assess for atrial enlargement and ventricular hypertrophy.
   a. Atrial enlargement (suggest lead $V_1$) (see Table 15-2)
   b. Ventricular hypertrophy (suggest lead $V_1$) (see Table 15-3)
5. Assess for heart blocks: RBBB, LBBB, and hemiblocks.
   a. Bundle branch blocks (suggest leads $V_1$, $V_2$ for RBBB and leads $V_5$, and $V_6$ for LBBB; see Table 15-4)
   b. Hemiblocks (suggest leads I, III; see Table 15-5)

*(6th step continued on page 130)*

**Figure 15-1   Calibration box and the continuous rhythm strip on the 12 lead ECG**

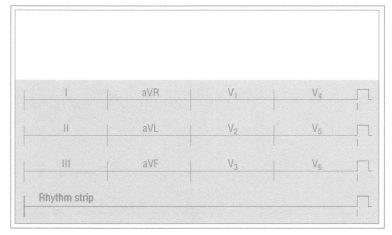

*Source*: From *12-Lead ECG: The Art of Interpretation*, courtesy of Tomas B. Garcia, MD.

**Figure 15-2    Electrical axis**

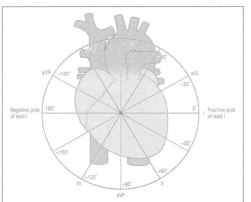

*Source*: From *12-Lead ECG: The Art of Interpretation*, courtesy of Tomas B. Garcia, MD.

**Table 15-1    Determine Electrical Axis (Suggest Leads I and II)**

|  | Lead I | Lead II |
|---|---|---|
| Normal | Upright | Upright |
| Left axis deviation (LAD) | Upright | Downward |
| Right axis deviation (RAD) | Downward | Upright |
| Extreme right axis | Downward | Downward |

**Table 15-2   Atrial Enlargement**

|  | Right Atrial Enlargement ($V_1$) (Figure 15-3) | Left Atrial Enlargement ($V_1$) (Figure 15-4) |
|---|---|---|
| P wave | Diphasic in $V_1$. The first half of the P wave is large and peaked (P wave > 2.5 mm or 0.25 mV in height). | Diphasic in $V_1$. The second half of the P wave is large, wide, and negative (P wave > 0.12 sec or 120 ms in duration). |

**Table 15-3   Ventricular Hypertrophy**

|  | Right Ventricular Hypertrophy ($V_1$) (Figure 15-5) | Left Ventricular Hypertrophy ($V_1$) (Figure 15-6 & 15-7) |
|---|---|---|
| QRS complex | Large R wave, small S wave in $V_1$ (positive) | Large S wave in $V_1$ (negative) and large R wave in $V_5$ or $V_6$ (S + R > 35 mm = LVH) |
| Axis deviation | Right axis deviation | Left axis deviation |
| R wave progression | Abnormal | Abnormal |

**Figure 15-3    Right atrial enlargement**

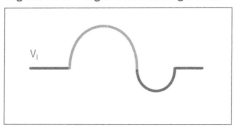

*Source*: From *12-Lead ECG: The Art of Interpretation*, courtesy of Tomas B. Garcia, MD.

**Figure 15-4    Left atrial enlargement**

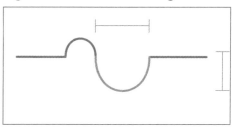

*Source*: From *12-Lead ECG: The Art of Interpretation*, courtesy of Tomas B. Garcia, MD.

**Figure 15-5    Right ventricular hypertrophy**

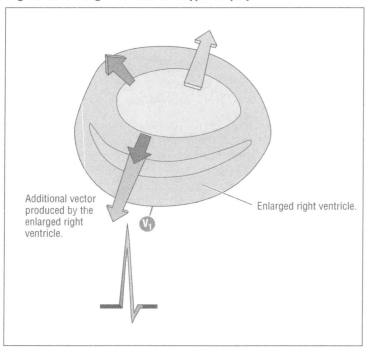

Additional vector produced by the enlarged right ventricle.

Enlarged right ventricle.

*Source*: From *12-Lead ECG: The Art of Interpretation*, courtesy of Tomas B. Garcia, MD.

**Figure 15-6    Measuring for left ventricular hypertrophy**

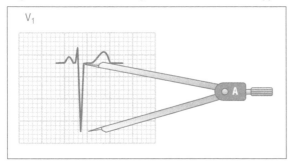

*Source*: From *12-Lead ECG: The Art of Interpretation*, courtesy of Tomas B. Garcia, MD.

**Figure 15-7    Left ventricular hypertrophy**

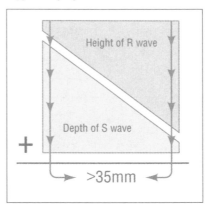

*Source*: From *12-Lead ECG: The Art of Interpretation*, courtesy of Tomas B. Garcia, MD.

**Table 15-4    Bundle Branch Blocks**

|  | RBBB (V$_1$, V$_2$)<br>(Figure 15-8) | LBBB (V$_5$, V$_6$)<br>(Figure 15-9) |
|---|---|---|
| QRS | $\geq$ 0.12 sec (120 ms) | $\geq$ 0.12 sec (120 ms) |
| QRS complex (R, R$^1$) | V$_1$, V$_2$ (can look like rabbit ears)<br>rsR$^1$ or rSR$^1$ | V$_5$, V$_6$ (broad, notched R waves)<br>rsR$^1$ or RR$^1$ |
| QRS in V$^1$ | Positive (upward) | Negative (downward) |
| Axis | Difficult to assess | Difficult to assess |

**Table 15-5    Hemiblocks**

|  | Anterior Hemiblock (I, III) (Figure 15-10) | Posterior Hemiblock (I, III) (Figure 15-11) |
|---|---|---|
| QRS | 0.10–0.12 sec | 0.10–0.12 seconds |
| QRS complex | Q in lead I; S (wide and deep) in lead III | S (wide and deep) in lead I; Q in lead III |
| Axis | Left axis deviation | Right axis deviation |

**Figure 15-8  EKG & RBBB**

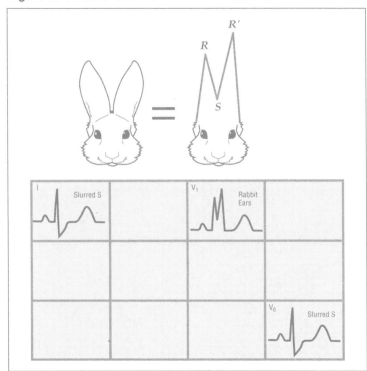

*Source*: From *12-Lead ECG: The Art of Interpretation*, courtesy of Tomas B. Garcia, MD.

**Figure 15-9  EKG & LBBB**

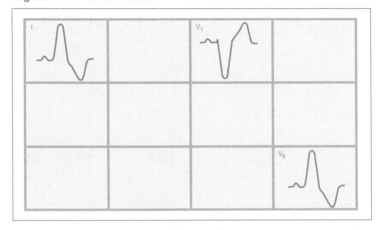

*Source*: From *12-Lead ECG: The Art of Interpretation*, courtesy of Tomas B. Garcia, MD.

**Figure 15-10   Anterior hemiblock**

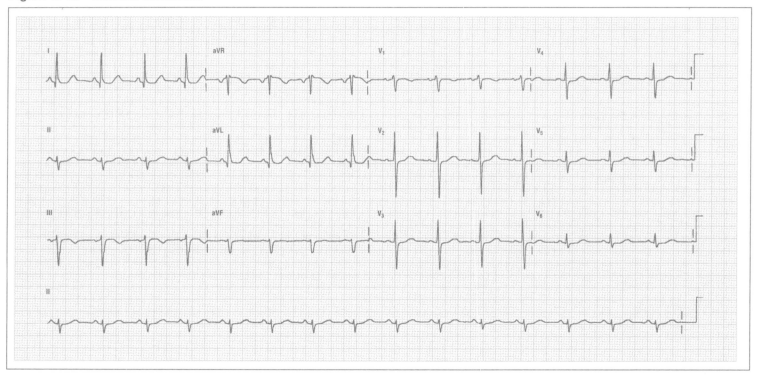

*Source*: From *12-Lead ECG: The Art of Interpretation*, courtesy of Tomas B. Garcia, MD.

**Figure 15-11    Posterior hemiblock**

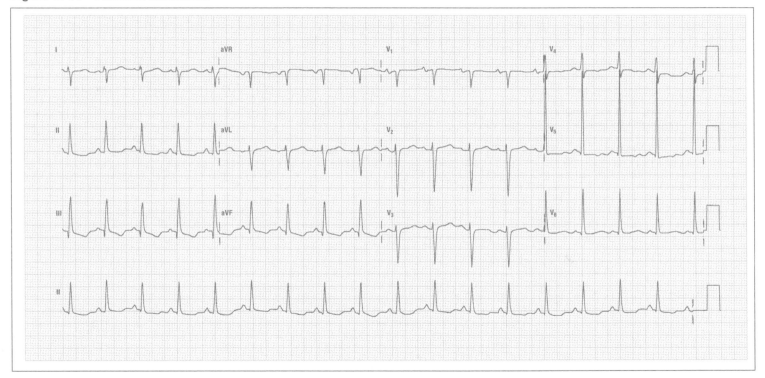

*Source*: From *12-Lead ECG: The Art of Interpretation*, courtesy of Tomas B. Garcia, MD.

6. Assess for area(s) of injury (ST segment elevation, ST segment depression, T wave inversion), ischemia (ST segment depression, T wave inversion), and infarction (Q waves) Please refer to the heading *Suggested Lead Sets* in this section.

a. ST segment elevation (injury; see Figure 15-12)

 i. A new or presumed new ST segment elevation greater than 1 mm or 0.1 mV at the J point in two contiguous precordial leads or two or more adjacent limb leads, and/or

 ii. ST segment elevation greater than or equal to 2 mm or 0.2 mV in men and greater than or equal to 1.5 mm or 0.15 mV in women in leads $V_1$–$V_3$ in the absence of left ventricular hypertrophy and left bundle branch block is classified as an ST segment elevation myocardial infarction (STEMI) (Thygesen, et al., 2007).

b. ST segment depression (injury/ischemia; see Figure 15-13)

 i. ST depression that is new or downsloping and is greater than or equal to 0.5 mm or 0.05 mV in two contiguous leads in the absence of left ventricular hypertrophy or left bundle branch block is classified as a non-ST-segment elevation myocardial infarction (NSTEMI) (Thygesen, et al., 2007).

 ii. ST depression, in the absence of a myocardial infarction, is indicative of ischemia.

c. T wave inversion (ischemia/injury; see Figure 15-14)

 i. T wave inversion with a depth greater than or equal to 1 mm or 0.1 mV in two contiguous leads with a prominent R wave or R:S ratio greater than 1 in the absence of left ventricular hypertrophy and left bundle branch block is classified as a non-ST-segment elevation myocardial infarction (NSTEMI) (ACC Clinical Data Standards, 2001; Thygesen, et al., 2007).

**Figure 15-12   Elevated ST segment**

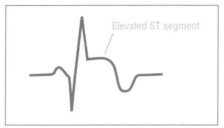

Elevated ST segment

*Source*: Porter, W. *Porter's pocket guide to emergency and critical care*. Jones and Bartlett Publishers.

*Note:* ST segment elevation associated with an acute myocardial infarction is convex or dome shaped.

Figure 15-13    ST depression

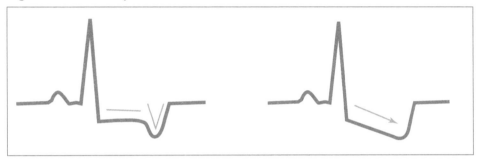

*Source*: From *12-Lead ECG: The Art of Interpretation*, courtesy of Tomas B. Garcia, MD.

Figure 15-14    T wave inversion

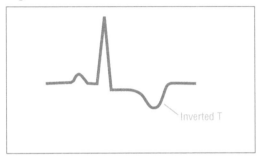

*Source*: Porter, W. *Porter's pocket guide to emergency and critical care*. Jones and Bartlett Publishers.

Figure 15-15    A pathologic Q wave

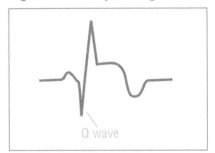

*Source*: Porter, W. *Porter's pocket guide to emergency and critical care*. Jones and Bartlett Publishers.

ii. T wave inversion, in the absence of a myocardial infarction, is indicative of myocardial ischemia.

d. Q wave (infarction/death of segment (s) of the heart muscle; see Figure 15-15)

i. A Q wave with a width greater than or equal to 0.04 sec or 40 ms and/or a height greater than or equal to one-fourth the R wave in at least two contiguous leads can be pathologic and indicative of a myocardial infarction (ACC/AHA/HRS, 2006).

## SUGGESTED LEAD SETS TO USE WHEN ASSESSING FOR INJURY, ISCHEMIA, AND/OR INFARCTION

- Lateral leads
  - I and $aV_L$ high lateral wall of the left ventricle
  - $V_5$ and $V_6$ low lateral wall of the left ventricle (see Figure 15-16)
    - Abnormality may indicate pathology on the lateral upper or lower wall of the left ventricle.
- Inferior leads
  - II, III, $aV_F$ (see Figure 15-17)

**Figure 15-16   Lateral wall injury**

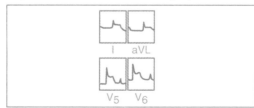

*Source*: Porter, W. *Porter's pocket guide to emergency and critical care*. Jones and Bartlett Publishers.

**Figure 15-17   Inferior wall injury**

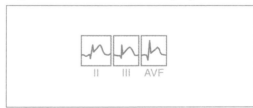

*Source*: Porter, W. *Porter's pocket guide to emergency and critical care*. Jones and Bartlett Publishers.

- ▪ Abnormality may indicate pathology on the inferior wall of the heart (also known as the diaphragmatic surface of the heart).
- Anterior leads
  - $V_1$, $V_2$, $V_3$, and $V_4$ (see Figure 15-18)
    - ▪ Abnormality may indicate pathology on the anterior wall of the left side of the heart.
    - ▪ Leads $V_1R–V_4R$ may indicate pathology on the anterior wall of the right side of the heart.
- Septal leads
  - $V_2$ and $V_3$
  - Abnormality may indicate pathology of the interventricular septum.

> **Injury to the Heart**
>
> Injury, ischemia, or infarction can occur in more than one area of the heart, such as:
>
> - Anterior and lateral
> - Anterior, septal, and lateral
> - Inferior and lateral

**Figure 15-18  Anterior wall injury**

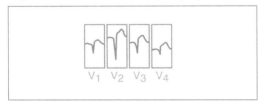

*Source*: Porter, W. *Porter's pocket guide to emergency and critical care*. Jones and Bartlett Publishers.

**Figure 15-19  Posterior (inferobasal) injury**

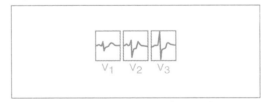

*Source*: Porter, W. *Porter's pocket guide to emergency and critical care*. Jones and Bartlett Publishers.

- Posterior (inferobasal)
  - $V_1$, $V_2$, $V_3$ reciprocal changes (see Figure 15-19)
    - Abnormality may indicate pathology of the posterior wall of the heart.
    - The EKG cannot take a direct picture of the posterior aspect of the heart, but it can indirectly show injury through reciprocal changes in leads $V_1$–$V_3$ because these leads mirror the posterior wall of the heart.
    - New guidelines suggest that the word "inferobasal" should replace the word "posterior" (Thygesen, et al., 2007, para. 27).

## OTHER CONDITIONS THAT CAN AFFECT THE EKG

Be on the lookout for other conditions that could affect the EKG (for the purposes of this handbook, only a few key EKG signs will be listed per condition). Patient history, family history, admitting diagnosis, clinical signs and symptoms, and other clinical diagnostic tools should be used, along with the EKG, to assist in making a diagnosis.

- Brugada syndrome (Brugada syndrome, n.d.; see Figure 15-20)
  - ST segment in leads $V_1$–$V_3$ is elevated, coved, and without reciprocal ST segment depression
  - RBBB, complete or incomplete
- Wellens syndrome (see Figure 15-21)
  - Marked T wave inversion in $V_2$ and $V_3$ (Conover, 2003)
- Wolff-Parkinson-White syndrome (Scheinman & Kaushik, 2003; see Figure 15-22)
  - Delta wave
  - Wide QRS
  - Short P-R interval
- Early repolarization (see Figure 15-23)
  - ST segment in the precordial leads is elevated, concave, looks like an upsloping smile, a fishhook, or a saddle (Pelter & Carey, 2007), and without reciprocal ST segment depression (Adams-Hamoda, et al., 2003; Nishimura & Kidd, 2003)

**Figure 15-20    Brugada ST elevation**

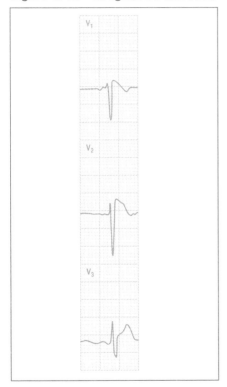

*Source*: From *Arrhythmia Recognition: The Art of Interpretation*, courtesy of Tomas B. Garcia, MD.

**Figure 15-21    Wellens Syndrome**

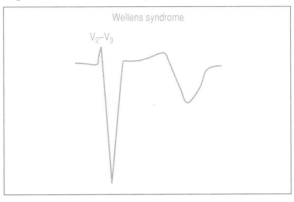

*Source*: Conover, M. B., *Understanding Electrocadiography*, St. Louis, 2003, Mosby.

**Figure 15-22   WPW and the delta wave**

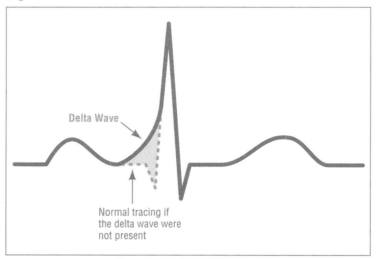

*Source*: From *12-Lead ECG: The Art of Interpretation*, courtesy of Tomas B. Garcia, MD.

**Figure 15-23   ST segment in early repolarization and pericarditis**

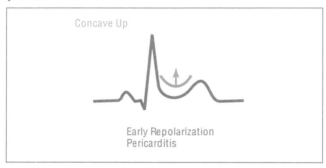

*Source*: From *12-Lead ECG: The Art of Interpretation*, courtesy of Tomas B. Garcia, MD.

- Acute pericarditis (see Figure 15-23)
  - ST segment elevation is widespread, concave, looks like an upsloping smile, a fishhook, or a saddle (Pelter & Carey, 2007), and without reciprocal ST segment depression (Adams-Hamoda, et al., 2003; Nishimura & Kidd, 2003)
  - P-R interval depression (often seen in leads II, III, VF) (Nishimura & Kidd, 2003)
- Conditions such as spontaneous pneumothorax, chronic obstructive pulmonary disease (Dubin, 2000), and pericardial effusion (Haberl, 2002–2005; see Figure 15-24)
  - Low voltage of the QRS
- Digitalis and other glycosides (Adams-Hamoda, et al., 2003; Dubin, 2000; see Figure 15-25)
  - ST segment depression that looks like a bowl or a soup ladle (Garcia & Holtz, 2001)
  - Flat, depressed, or inverted T waves
  - U waves can be more prominent
  - Shortened Q-T interval
  - J point depression
- Cyclic antidepressants
  - Prolongation of the PR, QRS, and QT/QTc (Garcia & Holtz, 2001; Soghoian, Doty, Maffei, & Connolly, 2006)
- Cocaine (Livingston, Mabie, & Ramanathan, 2000)
  - Prolongation of the PR, QRS, and QT/QTc
  - ST-T wave abnormalities
  - Pathologic Q waves
- Hypokalemia (see Figure 15-26)
  - U waves prominent as potassium values drop (Adams-Hamoda, et al., 2003; Dubin, 2000)
  - Flat or inverted T waves (Adams-Hamoda, et al., 2003)
- Hyperkalemia (see Figure 15-27)

**Figure 15-24   Low QRS voltage**

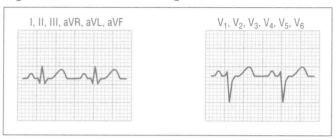

*Source*: From *12-Lead ECG: The Art of Interpretation*, courtesy of Tomas B. Garcia, MD.

**Figure 15-25   Segment and digitalis**

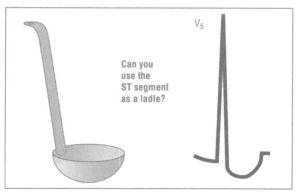

*Source*: From *12-Lead ECG: The Art of Interpretation*, courtesy of Tomas B. Garcia, MD.

**Figure 15-26   Hypokalemia and prominent U-waves**

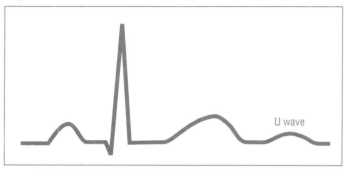

*Source*: From *12-Lead ECG: The Art of Interpretation*, courtesy of Tomas B. Garcia, MD.

**Figure 15-27    Hyperkalemia and tall, peaked, narrow T-waves**

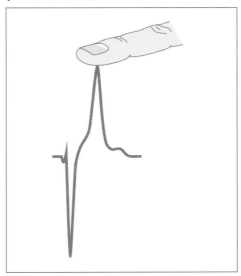

*Source*: From *12-Lead ECG: The Art of Interpretation*, courtesy of Tomas B. Garcia, MD.

**Figure 15-28    Hypocalcemia**

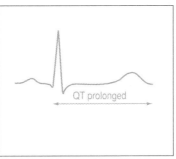

*Source*: From *12-Lead ECG: The Art of Interpretation*, courtesy of Tomas B. Garcia, MD.

- Tall, peaked, narrow T waves (Ganz, 2003)
- QRS widens as potassium values increase (Adams-Hamoda, et al., 2003; Dubin, 2000)
- P wave becomes wide, flat, or disappears (Dubin, 2000)
- Hypocalcemia (see Figure 15-28)
  - Prolongation of the Q-T interval (Dubin, 2000)
  - Prolongation of the ST segment (Adams-Hamoda, et al., 2003; Garcia & Holtz, 2001)
- Hypercalcemia (see Figure 15-29)
  - Shortened Q-T interval (Dubin, 2000)
  - Shortened ST segment (Adams-Hamoda, et al., 2003; Garcia & Holtz, 2001)
- Warning signs of impending torsades de pointes (see Figure 15-30)

**Figure 15-29   Hypercalcemia**

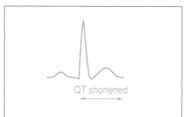

*Source*: From *12-Lead ECG: The Art of Interpretation*, courtesy of Tomas B. Garcia, MD.

**Figure 15-30   Progression of rhythm into Torsades**

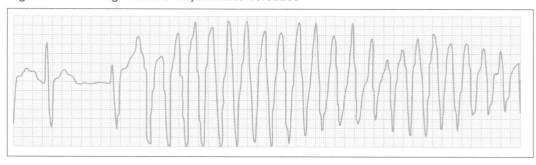

- – Prolongation of the QTc interval
- – Changes in height and polarity of the T wave (Keller, 2008)
- – Slower heart rates with pauses (Hebra, 1998)
- – New onset U wave (Hebra, 1998)

> *Note:* The Osborn wave is also known as the J wave, J deflection, or camel-hump sign, and it is a convex, upward deflection of the J point.

- Warning signs of cardiac instability associated with a propofol infusion
  - – ST segment elevation of $V_1$, $V_2$, and $V_3$ (Zaccheo & Bucher, 2008)
- Hypothermia (see Figure 15-31)
  - – Osborn wave prominent in leads II, III, $aV_F$, $V_5$, and $V_6$ (as hypothermia worsens, all leads become involved) (Bargout & Lucas, 2002)
- Pulmonary embolism
  - – T wave inversion in $V_1$–$V_4$ (Dubin, 2000; Shaughnessy, 2007)
  - – Transient complete or incomplete RBBB (Dubin, 2000)
- Subarachnoid hemorrhage and intracerebral bleed (see Figure 15-32)
  - – Prolongation of the QT/QTc (Bargout & Lucas, 2002; Keller, 2008)
  - – Deeply inverted T waves (Bargout & Lucas, 2002)
  - – Prominent U waves (Bargout & Lucas, 2002)
- Normal variants
  - – Healthy young men: Concave ST segment elevations 1–3 mm or 0.1–0.3 mV (most marked in $V_2$) (Bhatia & Kaul, 2007)
  - – Healthy patients (1–2%): ST segment depression (Ganz, 2003)
  - – Healthy patients (4%): T wave inversion (Ganz, 2003)
  - – A Q wave of any size is normal in leads III and $aV_R$ (Wagner & Lim, 2008a)

**Figure 15-31 Hypothermia and the Osborn or J wave**

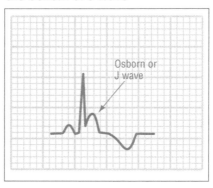

*Source*: From *12-Lead ECG: The Art of Interpretation*, courtesy of Tomas B. Garcia, MD.

**Figure 15-32 Deeply inverted T-waves associated with head bleeds**

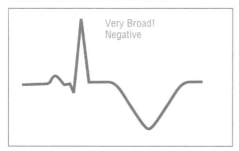

*Source*: From *12-Lead ECG: The Art of Interpretation*, courtesy of Tomas B. Garcia, MD.

# Rhythms

There are five categories of rhythms:

- Sinus: "I have a regular tempo but the beat is off at times."
- Escape: "Oh my goodness, it is late so I better add a beat."
- Premature: "Let me squeeze an early beat in here."
- Blocked: "I think I will slow down the beat."
- Tachyarrhythmias: "I think I will pump up the beat."

Ninety percent of patients with an acute myocardial infarction (MI) will have some form of rhythm abnormality. The most common arrhythmias after an MI are sinus tachycardia and premature ventricular beats and sinus bradycardia with inferior infarctions (Hebbar & Hueston, 2002).

*Note:* Although the information throughout this section is not all-inclusive, the goal is to provide the reader with enough information to assist in the understanding and interpretation of each rhythm. It is important to note, however, that while the rhythms will be presented in isolation from one another in this handbook, the rhythms can and are often combined in the clinical setting. Here are just a few examples: Sinus rhythm with a right bundle branch block, first degree heart block with occasional premature atrial beats, supraventricular tachycardia with a left bundle branch block, atrial fibrillation with occasional 3–4 beats runs of ventricular tachycardia, sinus tachycardia with atrial bigeminy, third degree heart block with occasional premature ventricular beats, etc.

Please note the following symbols (* or **) that will appear throughout this section:

* Unable to assess if the $V_1$ lead is not used for analysis. Most of the rhythms used in this handbook are not from the $V_1$ lead.

** Although the QT and QT c values should be included in routine analysis of the EKG, the values will not be measured in this section.

## SINUS RHYTHMS

*"I have a regular tempo but the beat is off at times."*

Sinus rhythms occur when the electrical impulse is initiated in the SA node and travels in a normal fashion down the electrical circuit of the heart. Drugs, disease, exercise, respiration, physical health, age, and condition of the sinus node can alter the rate of the sinus rhythm and the presentation of the rhythm on the EKG.

### Normal Sinus Rhythm

Normal sinus rhythm (see Figure 16-1) is the normal or natural rhythm of the heart that occurs when the electrical impulse travels from the SA node down through the Purkinje fibers at a rate of 60–100 beats per minute.

**Figure 16-1  Sinus Rhythm**

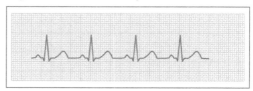

*Source*: Jackson, J. & Jackson, L. *Clinical nursing pocket guide*. Jones and Bartlett Publishers.

**Rate**
☒ Normal (60–100 beats per minute)
❑ Bradycardia (< 60 beats per minute)
❑ Tachycardia (> 100 beats per minute)

**Rhythm**
☒ Regular
❑ Irregular

**P waves**
☒ P wave occurs before each QRS complex
☒ P waves look the same in shape and size
❑ P waves in $V_1$ are monophasic, < 0.12 sec in duration, < 2.5 mm (0.25 mV) in height*
❑ P waves cannot be found

**P-R interval**
☒ Normal (0.12 sec to 0.20 sec)
❑ Short (< 0.12 sec)
❑ Long (> 0.20 sec)
❑ Cannot determine

**QRS complex**
☒ QRS complex occurs after each P wave
☒ QRS complexes look the same in shape and size
☒ QRS complex is normal (< 0.12 sec)
❑ QRS complex is wide (≥ 0.12 sec)

**QRS complex direction in $V_1$***
❑ Negative
❑ Positive
❑ Cannot determine

**Q-T interval\*\***
❑ Normal (≤ 0.40 sec)

**QTc\*\***
❑ Normal (men ≤ 0.44 sec, women ≤ 0.46 sec)
❑ Long or approaching the danger zone (> 0.50 sec)

## Sinus Bradycardia

Sinus bradycardia (see Figure 16-2) occurs when the electrical impulse travels from the SA node down through the Purkinje fibers at a rate less than 60 beats per minute while maintaining normal P wave morphology and a normal P-R interval.

**Figure 16-2   Sinus Bradycardia**

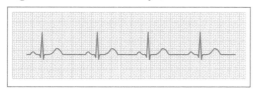

*Source*: Jackson, J. & Jackson, L. *Clinical nursing pocket guide*. Jones and Bartlett Publishers.

**Rate**
❑ Normal (60–100 beats per minute)
☒ Bradycardia (< 60 beats per minute)
❑ Tachycardia (> 100 beats per minute)

**Rhythm**
☒ Regular
❏ Irregular

**P waves**
☒ P wave occurs before each QRS complex
☒ P waves look the same in shape and size
❏ P waves in $V_1$ are monophasic, < 0.12 sec in duration, < 2.5 mm (0.25 mV) in height*
❏ P waves cannot be found

**P-R interval**
☒ Normal (0.12 sec to 0.20 sec)
❏ Short (< 0.12 sec)
❏ Long (> 0.20 sec)
❏ Cannot determine

**QRS complex**
☒ QRS complex occurs after each P wave
☒ QRS complexes look the same in shape and size
☒ QRS complex is normal (< 0.12 sec)
❏ QRS complex is wide (≥ 0.12 sec)

**QRS complex direction in $V_1$***
❏ Negative
❏ Positive
❏ Cannot determine

**Q-T interval\*\***
❑ Normal (≤ 0.40 sec)

**QTc\*\***
❑ Normal (men ≤ 0.44 sec, women ≤ 0.46 sec)
❑ Long or approaching the danger zone (> 0.50 sec)

• After an acute inferior myocardial infarction, 40% of patients can develop a sinus bradycardia (Hebbar & Hueston, 2002).
• Sinus bradycardia can be normal in some individuals, such as well-trained athletes. It also is normal during deep sleep cycles (American Heart Association, 2007d).
• Persistent heart rates less than 45 beats per minute in individuals who are not well-trained athletes and who are not taking medications to lower the rate are considered to be abnormal and may reflect disease to the SA node (American Heart Association, 2007d).

## Sinus Tachycardia

Sinus tachycardia (see Figure 16-3) occurs when the electrical impulse travels from the SA node down through the Purkinje fibers at a rate greater than 100 but less than 150 beats per minute in a nonexercising adult (Gilbert & Wagner, 2008a).

**Figure 16-3   Sinus Tachycardia**

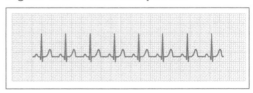

*Source*: Jackson, J. & Jackson, L. *Clinical nursing pocket guide*. Jones and Bartlett Publishers.

*Note:* In an adult, sinus tachycardia rarely exceeds 180 beats per minute (Scheinman & Kaushik, 2003).

## Rate
- ☐ Normal (60–100 beats per minute)
- ☐ Bradycardia (< 60 beats per minute)
- ☒ Tachycardia (> 100 beats per minute)

## Rhythm
- ☒ Regular
- ☐ Irregular

## P waves
- ☒ P wave occurs before each QRS complex
- ☒ P waves look the same in shape and size
- ☐ P waves in $V_1$ are monophasic, < 0.12 sec in duration, < 2.5 mm (0.25 mV) in height*
- ☐ P waves cannot be found

## P-R interval
- ☒ Normal (0.12 sec to 0.20 sec)
- ☐ Short (< 0.12 sec)
- ☐ Long (> 0.20 sec)
- ☐ Cannot determine

## QRS complex
- ☒ QRS complex occurs after each P wave
- ☒ QRS complexes look the same in shape and size
- ☒ QRS complex is normal (< 0.12 sec)
- ☐ QRS complex is wide (≥ 0.12 sec)

**QRS complex direction in V$_1$***
- ❏ Negative
- ❏ Positive
- ❏ Cannot determine

**Q-T interval****
- ❏ Normal (≤ 0.40 sec)

**QTc****
- ❏ Normal (men ≤ 0.44 sec, women ≤ 0.46 sec)
- ❏ Long or approaching the danger zone (> 0.50 sec)

## Sinus Arrhythmia

Sinus arrhythmia (see Figure 16-4) occurs when the electrical impulse travels from the SA node down through the Purkinje fiber at irregular intervals, causing variability in the sinus rate. Although a sinus arrhythmia can occur with "aging, postprandial hypotension, diabetes, alcoholic cardiomyopathy, acute inferior myocardial infarctions, increases in intracranial pressure, youth, and athleticism" (Conover, 2003, p. 52) and an increase in vagal tone, most sinus arrhythmias occur because of respiration, that is, the heart rate decreases with expiration and increases with inspiration.

**Rate**
- ☒ Normal (60–100 beats per minute)
- ❏ Bradycardia (< 60 beats per minute)
- ❏ Tachycardia (> 100 beats per minute)

**Rhythm**
- ❏ Regular
- ☒ Irregular

**Figure 16-4    Sinus Arrhythmia**

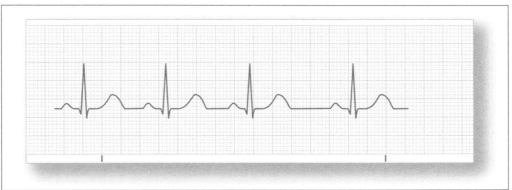

*Source*: From *Arrhythmia Recognition: The Art of Interpretation*, courtesy of Tomas B. Garcia, MD.

**P waves**
☒ P wave occurs before each QRS complex
☒ P waves look the same in shape and size
❑ P waves in $V_1$ are monophasic, < 0.12 sec in duration, < 2.5 mm (0.25 mV) in height*
❑ P waves cannot be found

**P-R interval**
☒ Normal (0.12 sec to 0.20 sec)
❑ Short (< 0.12 sec)

> *Note:* The P-R interval can change slightly with heart rate changes.

❑ Long (> 0.20 sec)
❑ Cannot determine

**QRS complex**
☒ QRS complex occurs after each P wave
☒ QRS complexes look the same in shape and size
☒ QRS complex is normal (< 0.12 sec)
❑ QRS complex is wide (≥ 0.12 sec)

**QRS complex direction in $V_1$\***
❑ Negative
❑ Positive
❑ Cannot determine

**Q-T interval\*\***
❑ Normal (≤ 0.40 sec)

**QTc\*\***
❑ Normal (men ≤ 0.44 sec, women ≤ 0.46 sec)
❑ Long or approaching the danger zone (> 0.50 sec)

## ESCAPE BEATS/RHYTHMS

*"Oh my goodness, it is late so I better add a beat."*

Escape beats/rhythms occur when the dominant or natural pacemaker of the heart is suppressed and an escape electrical focus emerges until the SA node resumes pacemaker control or until the escape rhythm is suppressed. Escape beats/rhythms can occur in the atria, in the atrioventricular junction, or in the ventricle. Other terms often associated with escape beats or rhythms are "idio-junctional," "idioventricular," and "back-up pacemakers."

## Atrial Escape Beat(s)/Rhythm

An atrial escape beat(s)/rhythm (see Figure 16-5) occurs when there is a pause of considerable length in the electrical circuit of the heart because the SA node fails to initiate and/or transmit an electrical impulse within a certain time frame. This pause causes an ectopic escape foci within the atria to assist the electrical circuit of the heart by initiating one or more electrical impulses until the SA node resumes pacemaker control of the heart or until the escape foci are suppressed. Because the atrial electrical impulse originates in the ectopic escape foci versus the sinus node, the P wave(s) will have a different morphology.

**Figure 16-5    Atrial escape beats**

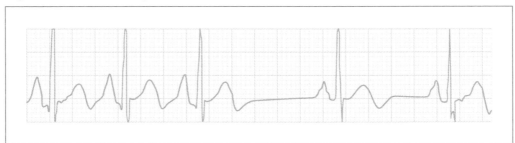

*Source*: From *Rapid Interpretation of EKG's* by Dale Dubin, MD with permission.

**Rate**
☒ Normal (60–100 beats per minute)
☒ Bradycardia (< 60 beats per minute)
☒ Tachycardia (> 100 beats per minute)

**Rhythm**
☒ Regular (if an atrial escape rhythm takes over; often see a pause before the escape foci kicks in)
☒ Irregular (if escape beat(s) occur; often see a pause before the escape foci kicks in)

**P waves**
☒ P wave occurs before each QRS complex (P waves will look different from the sinus P wave)
❑ P waves look the same in shape and size
❑ P waves in V1 are monophasic, < 0.12 seconds in duration, < 2.5 mm (0.25 mV) in height*
❑ P waves cannot be found

**P-R interval**
☒ Normal (0.12 sec to 0.20 sec)
❑ Short (< 0.12 sec)
❑ Long (> 0.20 sec)
❑ Cannot determine

**QRS complex**
☒ QRS complex occurs after each P wave
☒ QRS complexes look the same in shape and size
☒ QRS complex is normal (< 0.12 seconds)
❑ QRS complex is wide (≥ 0.12 sec)

## QRS complex direction in $V_1$*
❏ Negative
❏ Positive
❏ Cannot determine

## Q-T interval**
❏ Normal (≤ 0.40 sec)

## QTc**
❏ Normal (men ≤ 0.44 sec, women ≤ 0.46 sec)
❏ Long or approaching the danger zone (> 0.50 sec)

### Junctional or Idiojunctional Escape Beat (s) /Rhythm and Accelerated Junctional Rhythm

A junctional or idiojunctional escape beat(s)/rhythm (see Figure 16-6) occurs when there is a pause of considerable length in the electrical circuit of the heart because the SA node fails to initiate and/or transmit an electrical impulse within a certain time frame. If escape foci from the atria do not initiate an electrical impulse, this pause causes the pacemaker cells of the AV node to assume pacemaker control of the heart by initiating one or more electrical impulses until the SA node resumes pacemaker control or until the escape foci are suppressed. Because the electrical impulse originates in the AV node, there is no P wave (unless there is retrograde conduction, which will result in the P wave occurring immediately before, during, or after the QRS complex).

The pacing rate of the AV node is normally 40–60 beats per minute; however, if the rate accelerates to 60–100, the rhythm is called an accelerated junctional rhythm (see Figure 16-7).

## Rate
☒ Normal (60–100 beats per minute)
☒ Bradycardia (< 60 beats per minute)
❏ Tachycardia (> 100 beats per minute)

> If the AV node does not receive an electrical impulse within 1.0–1.5 sec after the SA node fires, the AV node will assume pacemaker control of the heart (American Heart Association, 2007a).

**Figure 16-6    Junctional escape beat**

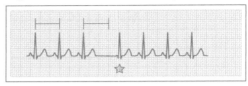

*Source*: Jackson, J. & Jackson, L. *Clinical nursing pocket guide*. Jones and Bartlett Publishers.

**Figure 16-7    Accelerated junctional rhythm**

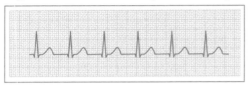

*Source*: Jackson, J. & Jackson, L. *Clinical nursing pocket guide*. Jones and Bartlett Publishers.

### Rhythm
☒ Regular (if an idiojunctional rhythm takes over; often see a pause before the escape foci kicks in)
☒ Irregular (if escape beat(s) occur; often see a pause before the escape foci kicks in)

### P waves
❑ P wave occurs before each QRS complex
❑ P waves look the same in shape and size
❑ P waves in V1 are monophasic, < 0.12 sec in duration, < 2.5 mm (0.25 mV) in height
☒ P waves cannot be found (P waves are often nonexistent or hidden; the best leads to see the P waves *if* they are present are leads II, III, and $aV_F$, where the P waves often have a negative deflection)

### P-R interval
❑ Normal (0.12 sec to 0.20 sec)
❑ Short (< 0.12 sec)
❑ Long (> 0.20 sec)
☒ Cannot determine

## QRS complex
❏ QRS complex occurs after each P wave
☒ QRS complexes look the same in shape and size
☒ QRS complex is normal (< 0.12 sec)
❏ QRS complex is wide (≥ 0.12 sec)

## QRS complex direction in $V_1$*
❏ Negative
❏ Positive
❏ Cannot determine

## Q-T interval**
❏ Normal (≤ 0.40 sec)

## QTc**
❏ Normal (men ≤ 0.44 sec, women ≤ 0.46 sec)
❏ Long or approaching the danger zone (> 0.50 sec)

### Ventricular or Idioventricular Escape Beat (s)/Rhythm and Accelerated Idioventricular Rhythm

A ventricular or idioventricular escape beat(s)/rhythm (see Figure 16-8) occurs when there is a pause of considerable length in the electrical circuit of the heart because the SA node *and* the AV node fail to initiate and/or transmit an electrical impulse within a certain time frame. If no escape foci occurs in the atria or in the AV node, this pause causes the pacemaker cells of the Purkinje fibers within the ventricle to assist the electrical circuit of the heart by initiating one or more electrical impulses until the SA node resumes pacemaker control of the heart or until the escape foci is suppressed. Because the electrical impulse originates in the ventricles, there is no P wave, and the QRS complex is wide and bizarre in appearance.

**Figure 16-8    Ventricular Escape**

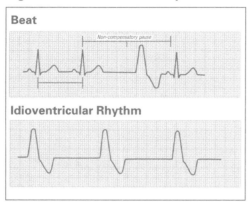

*Source*: Jackson, J. & Jackson, L. *Clinical nursing pocket guide*. Jones and Bartlett Publishers.

**Figure 16-9    Accelerated idioventricular rhythm**

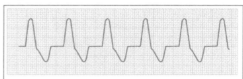

*Source*: Jackson, J. & Jackson, L. *Clinical nursing pocket guide*. Jones and Bartlett Publishers.

The pacing rate of the ventricular pacemaker cells is normally 20–40 beats per minute; however, if the rate is faster, it is called an accelerated idioventricular rhythm (see Figure 16-9). The usual rates associated with accelerated idioventricular rhythms are 75–100 beats per minute (American Heart Association, 2007f).

**Rate**
☒ Normal (60–100 beats per minute)
☒ Bradycardia (< 60 beats per minute)
❑ Tachycardia (> 100 beats per minute)

## Rhythm
☒ Regular (if a ventricular escape rhythm occurs; often see a pause before the escape foci kicks in)
☒ Irregular (if escape beat(s) occurs; often see a pause before the escape foci kicks in)

## P waves
❑ P wave occurs before each QRS complex
❑ P waves look the same in shape and size
❑ P waves in V1 are monophasic, < 0.12 sec in duration, < 2.5 mm (0.25 mV) in height*
☒ P waves cannot be found

## P-R interval
❑ Normal (0.12 sec to 0.20 sec)
❑ Short (< 0.12 sec)
❑ Long (> 0.20 sec)
☒ Cannot determine (no P waves)

## QRS complex
❑ QRS complex occurs after each P wave
❑ QRS complexes look the same in shape and size
❑ QRS complex is normal (< 0.12 sec)
☒ QRS complex is wide (≥ 0.12 sec; fusion beats can occur if the normal electrical circuit transmits an impulse to the ventricles at the same time the escape foci fires)

## QRS complex direction in $V_1$*
❑ Negative
❑ Positive
❑ Cannot determine

**Q-T interval**\*\*
❑ Normal (≤ 0.40 sec)

**QTc**\*\*
❑ Normal (men ≤ 0.44 sec, women ≤ 0.46 sec)

| |
|---|
| **What Is a Fusion Beat?** |
| A fusion beat is an abnormal beat that occurs when two beats from different pacemaker sites fuse at the same time. Example: A beat initiated by the SA node fuses at the same time with a beat initiated by the ventricle. |

- Accelerated idioventricular rhythm is usually intermittent and transient (American Heart Association, 2007f).
- After an acute myocardial infarction, 15-20% of patients can develop an accelerated idioventricular rhythm (Hebbar & Hueston, 2002).
- Reperfusion arrhythmias, which can occur when a previously occluded coronary artery is reopened, are often accelerated idioventricular rhythms (American Heart Association, 2007f).
- Slow idioventricular rhythms are also referred to as agonal rhythms.

## PREMATURE BEATS/RHYTHMS

*"Let me squeeze an early beat in here."*

Premature beats/rhythms occur when an irritable ectopic foci produces an electrical impulse that arrives early in the electrical circuit of the heart. Premature beats can occur in the atria, in the AV junction, or in the ventricles, and they can cause an abnormal beat or a rhythm that can override the normal electrical circuit and assume pacemaker control of the heart.

### Premature Atrial Beat

A premature atrial beat (see Figure 16-10), often referred to as a premature atrial complex (PAC), an atrial premature contraction (APC), or an atrial premature beat (APB), is a beat that occurs when an irritable ectopic electrical impulse from within the atria is initiated early in the electrical circuit of the heart. The premature beat can occur as an isolated beat(s), or it can lead to the initiation of a rhythm that can override the SA node and assume pacemaker control of the heart, that is, paroxysmal atrial tachycardia (this will be covered in the Tachyarrhythmia section). Because the atrial electrical impulse originates outside of the SA node, the P wave(s) will have a different morphology from the normal sinus P wave and it can be hidden in the ST segment or the T wave of the preceding complex. .

Caffeine, stress, smoking, amphetamines, cocaine, excess digitalis, and an imbalance between the sympathetic and parasympathetic systems are a few causes that can stimulate an irritable focus within the atria or the AV junction, producing a premature atrial beat(s) or a premature junctional beat(s) (Dubin, 1996).

## Rate
☒ Normal (60–100 beats per minute; rate depends on the underlying rhythm)
☒ Bradycardia (< 60 beats per minute)
☒ Tachycardia (> 100 beats per minute)

## Rhythm
❑ Regular
☒ Irregular

**Figure 16-10    Premature Atrial Beat**

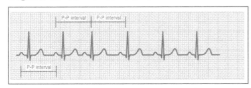

*Source*: Jackson, J. & Jackson, L. *Clinical nursing pocket guide*. Jones and Bartlett Publishers.

## P waves
☒ P wave occurs before each QRS complex (the P wave may be hidden in the ST segment or T wave of the preceding complex)
☒ P waves look the same in shape and size (the P waves associated with the premature atrial beat may be different in size and shape from the normal sinus P wave)
❏ P waves in $V_1$ are monophasic, < 0.12 sec in duration, < 2.5 mm (0.25 mV) in height*
❏ P waves cannot be found

## P-R interval
☒ Normal (0.12 sec to 0.20 sec; the P-R interval can vary with the premature atrial beat)
❏ Short (< 0.12 sec)
❏ Long (> 0.20 sec)
❏ Cannot determine

## QRS complex
☒ QRS complex occurs after each P wave
☒ QRS complexes look the same in shape and size
☒ QRS complex is normal (< 0.12 sec)
❏ QRS complex is wide (≥ 0.12 sec)

## QRS complex direction in $V_1$*
❏ Negative
❏ Positive
❏ Cannot determine

## Q-T interval**
❏ Normal (≤ 0.40 sec)

## QTc**
❑ Normal (men ≤ 0.44 sec, women ≤ 0.46 sec)
❑ Long or approaching the danger zone (> 0.50 sec)

• Premature atrial beats are more common than premature junctional beats.

## Premature Junctional Beat

A premature junctional beat (see Figure 16-11), often referred to as a premature junctional contraction (PJC), a junctional premature contraction (JPC), or a junctional premature beat (JPB), is a beat that occurs when an irritable ectopic electrical impulse from within the AV junction (the AV junction includes the AV node and the His Bundle) is initiated early in the electrical circuit of the heart. The premature beat can occur as an isolated beat(s), or it can lead to the initiation of a rhythm that can override the SA node and assume pacemaker control of the heart, that is, paroxysmal junctional ectopic tachycardia (this will be covered in the Tachyarrhythmia section). Because the electrical impulse originates in the AV junction, there is no P wave (unless there is retrograde conduction, which will result in the P wave occurring immediately before, during, or after the QRS complex).

**Figure 16-11    Premature Junctional Beat**

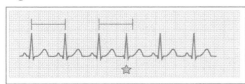

Source: Jackson, J. & Jackson, L. *Clinical nursing pocket guide*. Jones and Bartlett Publishers.

**Rate**

☒ Normal (60–100 beats per minute; rate depends on the underlying rhythm)
☒ Bradycardia (< 60 beats per minute)
☒ Tachycardia (> 100 beats per minute)

**Rhythm**

❏ Regular
☒ Irregular

**P waves**

❏ P wave occurs before each QRS complex
❏ P waves look the same in shape and size
❏ P waves in V1 are monophasic, < 0.12 sec in duration, < 2.5 mm (0.25 mV) in height
☒ P waves cannot be found (P waves are often nonexistent or hidden; the best leads to see the P waves if they are present are leads II, III, and $aV_F$, where the P waves often have a negative deflection)

**P-R interval**

❏ Normal
❏ Short (< 0.12 sec)
❏ Long (> 0.20 sec)
☒ Cannot determine

**QRS complex**

❏ QRS complex occurs after each P wave
☒ QRS complexes look the same in shape and size
☒ QRS complex is normal (< 0.12 sec)
❏ QRS complex is wide (≥ 0.12 sec)

## QRS complex direction in $V_1$*
☐ Negative
☐ Positive
☐ Cannot determine

## Q-T interval**
☐ Normal (≤ 0.40 sec)

## QTc**
☐ Normal (men ≤ 0.44 sec, women ≤ 0.46 sec)
☐ Long or approaching the danger zone (> 0.50 sec)

## Premature Ventricular Beat

A premature ventricular beat (PVB) (see Figure 16-12), often referred to as a premature ventricular contraction (PVC), a ventricular premature contraction (VPC), or a ventricular prema-

---

**Bigeminy, Trigeminy, Quadrigeminy**

Bigeminy, trigeminy, and quadrigeminy are abnormal rhythms that have a regularly occurring pattern of normal beats combined with an abnormal and often premature atrial, junctional, or ventricular beat:

- Bigeminy: A regularly occurring pattern of beats that includes a normal beat followed by an abnormal, premature beat (see Figure 16-13).
- Trigeminy: A regularly occurring pattern of beats that includes two normal beats followed by an abnormal, premature beat.
- Quadrigeminy: A regularly occurring pattern of beats that includes three normal beats followed by an abnormal, premature beat.

---

ture beat (VPB), is a beat that occurs when an irritable ectopic electrical impulse from within the ventricle is initiated early in the electrical circuit of the heart. The premature beat can occur as an isolated beat(s), or it can lead to the initiation of a rhythm that can override the SA node and assume pacemaker control of the heart, that is, paroxysmal ventricular tachycardia (this will be covered in the Tachyarrhythmia section). Because the electrical impulse originates in the ventricles, there is no P wave, and the QRS complex is wide and bizarre in appearance.

### Rate
☒ Normal (60–100 beats per minute; rate depends on the underlying rhythm)
☒ Bradycardia (< 60 beats per minute)
☒ Tachycardia (> 100 beats per minute)

## Figure 16-12    Premature Ventricular Beat

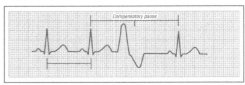

*Source*: Jackson, J. & Jackson, L. *Clinical nursing pocket guide*. Jones and Bartlett Publishers.

## Figure 16-13    Ventricular Bigemi

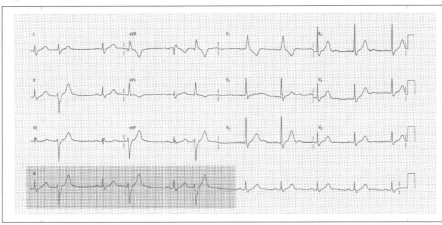

*Source*: From *12-Lead ECG: The Art of Interpretation*, courtesy of Tomas B. Garcia, MD.

**Rhythm**
❑ Regular
☒ Irregular

**P waves**
❑ P wave occurs before each QRS complex
❑ P waves look the same in shape and size
❑ P waves in V1 are monophasic, < 0.12 sec in duration, < 2.5 mm (0.25 mV) in height*
☒ P waves cannot be found

**P-R interval**
❑ Normal
❑ Short (< 0.12 sec)
❑ Long (> 0.20 sec)
☒ Cannot determine

## QRS complex
☐ QRS complex occurs after each P wave
☐ QRS complexes look the same in shape and size
☐ QRS complex is normal (< 0.12 sec)
☒ QRS complex is wide (≥ 0.12 sec; PVBs are wide, bizarre, and often followed by a compensatory pause)

## QRS complex direction in $V_1$*
☐ Negative
☐ Positive
☐ Cannot determine

## Q-T interval**
☐ Normal (≤ 0.40 sec)

## QTc**
Normal (men ≤ 0.44 sec, women ≤ 0.46 sec)
Long or approaching the danger zone (> 0.50 sec)

*Note:* A compensatory pause is a pause that compensates for the early arrival of the premature beat. It occurs after a premature beat and the pause enables the normal sinus rate to reset itself and get back on schedule (See figure 16-12). A non-compensatory pause is a pause that does not compensate for the early arrival of the premature beat. It occurs after a premature beat but does not enable the normal sinus rate to reset itself. Instead, the rate is completely reset and a new schedule is established (Garcia & Holtz, 2001).

- PVBs are usually followed by a compensatory pause.
- PVBs can be wide and bizarre in shape because they originate in the ventricle.
- The T waves associated with PVBs are opposite in direction from the normal QRS (Hebbar & Hueston, 2002).
- Three or more consecutive PVBs is defined as ventricular tachycardia.
- PVBs are common after a myocardial infarction (Hebbar & Hueston, 2002).
- PVBs are often considered to be markers of reperfusion when a previously occluded coronary artery is reopened (Conover, 2003).

## BLOCKED RHYTHMS

*"I think I will slow down the beat."*

Heart blocks occur when there is a block in the electrical circuit of the heart that leads to (1) a prolongation in the transmission of the electrical impulse, (2) a missed electrical impulse, or (3) no electrical impulse. Heart blocks can occur in the SA node, the AV node, the bundle branches, the fascicles, and the Purkinjes.

### Sinus Arrest/Sinus Pause

A sinus arrest or sinus pause (see Figure 16-14) occurs when the SA node fails to initiate an electrical impulse. This results in a sudden absence of sinus activity on the EKG until the SA node resumes control or until a back-up pacemaker from the atria, the AV junction, or the ventricle assumes control (Mishell & Goldschlager, 2003).

**Figure 16-14   Sinus Arrest/Sinus Pause**

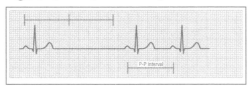

*Source*: Jackson, J. & Jackson, L. *Clinical nursing pocket guide*. Jones and Bartlett Publishers.

**Rate**

☒ Normal (60–100 beats per minute; rate may vary)
☒ Bradycardia (< 60 beats per minute)
❑ Tachycardia (> 100 beats per minute)

## Rhythm
❏ Regular
☒ Irregular (the SA node fails to initiate electrical activity)

## P waves
☒ P wave occurs before each QRS complex
☒ P waves look the same in shape and size (the P wave will look different if an escape beat/rhythm takes over pacemaker control of the heart)
❏ P waves in V1 are monophasic, < 0.12 sec in duration, < 2.5 mm (0.25 mV) in height*
❏ P waves cannot be found

## P-R interval
☒ Normal (0.12 sec to 0.20 sec)
❏ Short (< 0.12 sec)
❏ Long (> 0.20 sec)
❏ Cannot determine

## QRS complex
☒ QRS complex occurs after each P wave
☒ QRS complexes look the same in shape and size
☒ QRS complex is normal (< 0.12 sec)
❏ QRS complex is wide (≥ 0.12 sec)

## QRS complex direction in $V_1$*
❏ Negative
❏ Positive
❏ Cannot determine

## Q-T interval**
❑ Normal (≤ 0.40 sec)

## QTc**
❑ Normal (men ≤ 0.44 sec, women ≤ 0.46 sec)
❑ Long or approaching the danger zone (> 0.50 sec)

- A sinus pause less than or equal to 3 sec in an asymptomatic athlete usually does not require further evaluation or treatment (Hebbar & Hueston, 2002). The pause in athletes can be attributed to a high degree of vagal tone.
- Patients can become symptomatic if the heart rate is not adequate to maintain cardiac output.

## Sinus Block (Sinus Exit Block)
A sinus block (or sinus exit block) (see Figure 16-15) occurs when the SA node initiates an electrical impulse, but the impulse is blocked from conducting through the normal circuit. This results in a loss of sinus activity on the EKG until the SA node resumes control. If the SA node is too slow in resuming control, the back-up pacemaker sites in the atria, the AV junction, or the ventricle can assume pacemaker control of the heart (Mishell & Goldschlager, 2003).

**Figure 16-15    Sinus Block**

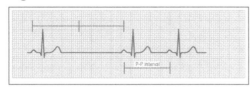

*Source*: Jackson, J. & Jackson, L. *Clinical nursing pocket guide*. Jones and Bartlett Publishers.

## Rate
☒ Normal (60–100 beats per minute; rate may vary)
☒ Bradycardia (< 60 beats per minute)
❑ Tachycardia (> 100 beats per minute)

## Rhythm
❑ Regular
☒ Irregular (the SA node initiates electrical activity but the electrical activity is blocked)

## P waves
☒ P wave occurs before each QRS complex
☒ P waves look the same in shape and size (the P wave will look different if an escape beat takes over pacemaker control of the heart)
❑ P waves in V1 are monophasic, < 0.12 sec in duration, < 2.5 mm (0.25 mV) in height*
❑ P waves cannot be found

## P-R interval
☒ Normal (0.12 sec to 0.20 sec)
❑ Short (< 0.12 sec)
❑ Long (> 0.20 sec)
❑ Cannot determine

## QRS complex
☒ QRS complex occurs after each P wave
☒ QRS complexes look the same in shape and size
☒ QRS complex is normal (< 0.12 sec)
❑ QRS complex is wide (≥ 0.12 sec)

**QRS complex direction in V₁***

❑ Negative
❑ Positive
❑ Cannot determine

**Q-T interval****

❑ Normal (≤ 0.40 sec)

**QTc****

❑ Normal (men ≤ 0.44 sec, women ≤ 0.46 sec)
❑ Long or approaching the danger zone (> 0.50 sec)

- Patients can become symptomatic if the heart rate is not adequate to maintain cardiac output.

> The difference between a sinus arrest/sinus pause and a sinus block is determined by what is happening in the SA node:
>
> - Sinus arrest/sinus pause–SA node is arrested and does not initiate an impulse
> - Sinus block–SA node initiates an impulse but is unable to transmit the impulse

### Sick Sinus Syndrome

Sick sinus syndrome (see Figure 16-16), also referred to as sinus node dysfunction, occurs when the SA node is "sick" and is unable to fire a consistent and regular electrical impulse. This condition causes marked sinus bradycardia, sinus arrest, sinus block, and, in some cases, a bradycardia–tachycardia syndrome (the heart speeds up and slows down) and paroxysmal episodes of atrial fibrillation and/or atrial flutter. Because the remainder of the electrical circuit is often sick in sick sinus syndrome, there is often no backup from the other pacemaker sites in the atria, the AV junction, or the ventricles.

**Rate**

☒ Normal (60–100 beats per minute; rates may vary-rhythm can speed up and slow down)
☒ Bradycardia (< 60 beats per minute)
☒ Tachycardia (> 100 beats per minute)

**Figure 16-16    Sick Sinus Syndrome**

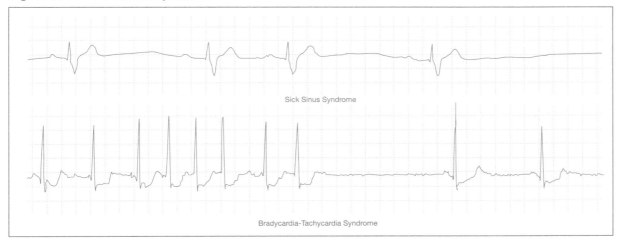

Sick Sinus Syndrome

Bradycardia-Tachycardia Syndrome

*Source*: From *Rapid Interpretation of EKG's* by Dale Dubin, MD with permission.

**Rhythm**
❑ Regular
☒ Irregular

**P waves**
☒ P wave occurs before each QRS complex (except if the patient is having episodes of atrial fibrillation or atrial flutter)
☒ P waves look the same in shape and size
❑ P waves in V1 are monophasic, < 0.12 sec in duration, < 2.5 mm (0.25 mV) in height*
❑ P waves cannot be found

**P-R interval**
☒ Normal (0.12 sec to 0.20 sec; if P waves are present)
❑ Short (< 0.12 sec)
☒ Long (> 0.20 sec)
❑ Cannot determine

**QRS complex**
☒ QRS complex occurs after each P wave (if P waves are present)
☒ QRS complexes look the same in shape and size
☒ QRS complex is normal (< 0.12 sec)
❑ QRS complex is wide (≥ 0.12 sec)

**QRS complex direction in $V_1$\***
❑ Negative
❑ Positive
❑ Cannot determine

**Q-T interval\*\***
❑ Normal (≤ 0.40 sec)

**QTc\*\***
❑ Normal (men ≤ 0.44 sec, women ≤ 0.46 sec)
❑ Long or approaching the danger zone (> 0.50 sec)

- "25% to 30% of patients with sinus node dysfunction have evidence of AV block and bundle branch block" (Mishell & Goldschlager, 2003, p. 534).
- The bradycardia–tachycardia phenomenon often occurs with sick sinus syndrome and can be a precursor to the development of chronic atrial fibrillation (Conover, 2003).

## First-Degree Heart Block

First-degree heart block (see Figure 16-17) is defined as abnormal prolongation of the P-R interval (P-R interval > 0.20 sec). Although the P-R interval is prolonged, conduction of the electrical impulse to the ventricles is normal.

**Figure 16-17    First Degree Heart Block**

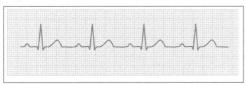

*Source*: Jackson, J. & Jackson, L. *Clinical nursing pocket guide*. Jones and Bartlett Publishers.

### Rate
☒ Normal (60–100 beats per minute; rates may vary)
☒ Bradycardia (< 60 beats per minute)
☒ Tachycardia (> 100 beats per minute)

### Rhythm
☒ Regular
❑ Irregular

### P waves
☒ P wave occurs before each QRS complex
☒ P waves look the same in shape and size

❏ P waves in V1 are monophasic, < 0.12 sec in duration, < 2.5 mm (0.25 mV) in height*
❏ P waves cannot be found

**P-R interval**
❏ Normal (0.12 sec to 0.20 sec)
❏ Short (< 0.12 sec)
☒ Long (> 0.20 sec)
❏ Cannot determine

**QRS complex**
☒ QRS complex occurs after each P wave
☒ QRS complexes look the same in shape and size
☒ QRS complex is normal (< 0.12 sec)
❏ QRS complex is wide (≥ 0.12 sec)

**QRS complex direction in $V_1$***
❏ Negative
❏ Positive
❏ Cannot determine

**Q-T interval****
❏ Normal (≤ 0.40 sec)

**QTc****
❏ Normal (men ≤ 0.44 sec, women ≤ 0.46 sec)
❏ Long or approaching the danger zone (> 0.50 sec)

• After acute inferior myocardial infarction, "15%" of patients can develop a first-degree heart block (Hebbar & Hueston, 2002, p. 2495).

## Type I Second-Degree Heart Block

Type I second-degree heart block (see Figure 16-18), also referred to as Mobitz type I or Wenckebach AV block, is characterized by a progressive prolongation of the P-R interval until one P wave does not conduct a beat and this produces a pause in the electrical circuit. This progressive prolongation of the P-R interval usually occurs as a group that can repeat itself and can vary, that is, 2:1, 3:2, 4: 3, etc. The following example would be referred to as a 4:3 Type I Second-Degree Heart Block or Wenckebach = 4 P waves and 3 QRS complexes:

PR–interval followed by a QRS complex
PR—interval followed by a QRS complex
PR——interval followed by a QRS complex
PR interval (*no* QRS complex)

**Rate**
☒ Normal (60–100 beats per minute)
☒ Bradycardia (< 60 beats per minute)
❑ Tachycardia (> 100 beats per minute)

**Figure 16-18    Type 1 Second-Degree Heart Block (3:2)**

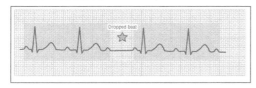

*Source*: Jackson, J. & Jackson, L. *Clinical nursing pocket guide*. Jones and Bartlett Publishers.

**Rhythm**
- ☐ Regular
- ☒ Irregular

**P waves**
- ☒ P wave occurs before each QRS complex
- ☒ P waves look the same in shape and size
- ☐ P waves in V1 are monophasic, < 0.12 sec in duration, < 2.5 mm (0.25 mV) in height*
- ☐ P waves cannot be found

**P-R interval**
- ☒ Normal (0.12 sec to 0.20 sec; P-R interval progressively lengthens until there is a missed beat, then the cycle or grouping repeats itself)
- ☐ Short (< 0.12 sec)
- ☐ Long (> 0.20 sec)
- ☐ Cannot determine

**QRS complex**
- ☐ QRS complex occurs after each P wave
- ☒ QRS complexes look the same in shape and size
- ☒ QRS complex is normal (< 0.12 sec)
- ☐ QRS complex is wide (≥ 0.12 sec)

**QRS complex direction in $V_1$\***
- ☐ Negative
- ☐ Positive
- ☐ Cannot determine

---

**Reversible Causes of AV Blocks**

Reversible causes of AV blocks are as follows (ACC/AHA/HRS, 2008):

- Electrolyte imbalances
- Drug toxicity
- Lyme disease
- Transient increases in vagal tone
- Hypothermia
- Inflammation near the AV node after surgery
- Hypoxia associated with sleep apnea
- Neurologic conditions
- Normal physiological AV block in the presence of SVT

**Q-T interval\*\***
- ❏ Normal (≤ 0.40 sec)

**QTc\*\***
- ❏ Normal (men ≤ 0.44 sec, women ≤ 0.46 sec)
- ❏ Long or approaching the danger zone (> 0.50 sec)

- There is often a shorter P-R interval after the nonconducted QRS beat.

- After an acute inferior myocardial infarction, "10%" of patients can develop a Mobitz type I block (Hebbar & Hueston, 2002, p. 2495).

### Type II Second-Degree Heart Block

Type II second-degree heart block (see Figure 16-19), also referred to as Mobitz type II, is characterized by sporadic nonconducted sinus P waves, that is:

### *Mobitz II Drops a Q out of the Blue*

The SA node initiates an electrical impulse and transmits the impulse to the AV node, but there is an intermittent conduction of the impulse through the ventricular conduction system because of disease or damage (see Figure 16-23 later in this section).

**Rate**
- ☒ Normal (60–100 beats per minute)
- ☒ Bradycardia (< 60 beats per minute)
- ❏ Tachycardia (> 100 beats per minute)

**Rhythm**
- ❏ Regular
- ☒ Irregular

**Figure 16-19    Type 11 Second-Degree Heart Block**

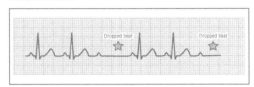

*Source*: Jackson, J. & Jackson, L. *Clinical nursing pocket guide*. Jones and Bartlett Publishers.

## P waves
☒ P wave occurs before each QRS complex
☒ P waves look the same in shape and size
❏ P waves in V1 are monophasic, < 0.12 sec in duration, < 2.5 mm (0.25 mV) in height*
❏ P waves cannot be found

## P-R interval
☒ Normal (0.12 sec to 0.20 sec; a normal P-R interval is a key identifier of this rhythm)
❏ Short (< 0.12 sec)
❏ Long (> 0.20 sec)
❏ Cannot determine

## QRS complex
❏ QRS complex occurs after each P wave
☒ QRS complexes look the same in shape and size
☒ QRS complex is normal (< 0.12 sec; if the level of the block is above the Bundle of His)
☒ QRS complex is wide (≥ 0.12 sec; if the level of the block is below the Bundle of His)

**QRS complex direction in $V_1$\***
❑ Negative
❑ Positive
❑ Cannot determine

**Q-T interval\*\***
❑ Normal ($\leq$ 0.40 sec)

**QTc\*\***
❑ Normal (men $\leq$ 0.44 sec, women $\leq$ 0.46 sec)
❑ Long or approaching the danger zone (> 0.50 sec)

---

### Fixed P-R Interval and Type II Heart Block

The fixed P-R interval is one characteristic that can assist in the differentiation of a type II second-degree heart block from a type I second-degree heart block and a third-degree heart block.

---

* Key identifiers of this rhythm are as follows:
  - The P-R interval is normal and fixed.
  - Missing QRS beats are preceded by a regular, punctual P wave.
  - Missing QRS beats are never preceded by a premature P wave (Dubin, 1996).
  - The P wave:QRS complex ratio can assist in the identification of the severity of the heart block, that is, 4:1 and 3:1 ratios are more severe and sometimes referred to as "advanced Mobitz II AV blocks" (Dubin, 1996, p. 173).

## Third-Degree Heart Block

Third-degree heart block (see Figure 16-20), also referred to as complete heart block, occurs when the sinus node initiates an electrical impulse, but the impulse is blocked from reaching the ventricles. The ventricles, therefore, initiate their own electrical impulse at a slower rate than that of the atrial rate. This is referred to as AV dissociation because the atria and the ventricles are working completely independent of each other.

**Figure 16-20    Third-Degree Heart Block**

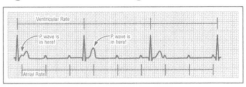

*Source*: Jackson, J. & Jackson, L. *Clinical nursing pocket guide*. Jones and Bartlett Publishers.

**The QRS Complex and Heart Blocks**

The width of the QRS complex will be determined by where the level of the block is in the intraventricular conduction system:

- If the level of the block is above the His bundle, the QRS complex will often be narrow or normal in appearance.
- If the level of the block is below the His bundle, the QRS complex will often be wide and bizarre in appearance.

**Rate**
- ❑ Normal (60–100 beats per minute)
- ☒ Bradycardia (< 60 beats per minute)
- ❑ Tachycardia (> 100 beats per minute)

**Rhythm**
- ☒ Regular (the P wave and the QRS are regular, but the QRS is not associated with the P wave)
- ❑ Irregular

**P waves**
- ❑ P wave occurs before each QRS complex
- ☒ P waves look the same in shape and size (but some are fused into the QRS or the T wave)
- ❑ P waves in V1 are monophasic, < 0.12 sec in duration, < 2.5 mm (0.25 mV) in height*
- ❑ P waves cannot be found

**P-R interval**
- ❑ Normal (0.12 sec to 0.20 sec)
- ❑ Short (< 0.12 sec)
- ❑ Long (> 0.20 sec)
- ☒ Cannot determine

> *Note:* A third-degree heart block can be missed because, at a quick glance, there can appear to be an association between the P wave and the QRS complex. This is one reason why a step by step analysis should be used when interpreting each rhythm.

**QRS complex**
- ❑ QRS complex occurs after each P wave
- ☒ QRS complexes look the same in shape and size (unless the P wave is fused into the QRS)
- ☒ QRS complex is normal (< 0.12 sec; if the level of the block is above the His Bundle)
- ☒ QRS complex is wide (≥ 0.12 sec; if the level of the block is below the His Bundle )

**QRS complex direction in $V_1$***
- ❑ Negative
- ❑ Positive
- ❑ Cannot determine

**Q-T interval****
- ❑ Normal (≤ 0.40 sec)

**QTc****
- ❑ Normal (men ≤ 0.44 sec, women ≤ 0.46 sec)
- ❑ Long or approaching the danger zone (> 0.50 sec)

- Third-degree heart block is often preceded by a bifasicular block.
- Syncope along with a transient third-degree heart block increases the risk of sudden death (ACC/AHA/HRS, 2008).

## Right Bundle Branch Block

A right bundle branch block (RBBB; see Figure 16-21) is a delay in the transmission of the electrical impulse from the right bundle branch to the ventricle. The delay occurs as the electrical impulse meets a block in the right bundle, causing the electrical impulse to move slowly around the block through the surrounding muscle of the heart. While there is a delay in the transmission of the impulse down the right bundle, there is regular rapid transmission of the impulse down the left bundle (if the left bundle is working appropriately). This asynchronous transmission of impulses results in depolarization of the left ventricle before the right ventricle.(Refer back to Section 6, Right Bundle Branch Block).

### Rate
☒ Normal (60–100 beats per minute; rate depends on the underlying rhythm)
☒ Bradycardia (< 60 beats per minute)
☒ Tachycardia (> 100 beats per minute)

### Rhythm
☒ Regular
☒ Irregular

### P waves
☒ P wave occurs before each QRS complex
☒ P waves look the same in shape and size
❑ P waves in V1 are monophasic, < 0.12 sec in duration, < 2.5 mm (0.25 mV) in height*
❑ P waves cannot be found

### P-R interval
☒ Normal (0.12 sec to 0.20 sec)
❑ Short (< 0.12 sec)
❑ Long (> 0.20 sec)
❑ Cannot determine

**Figure 16-21    Right Bundle Branch Block**

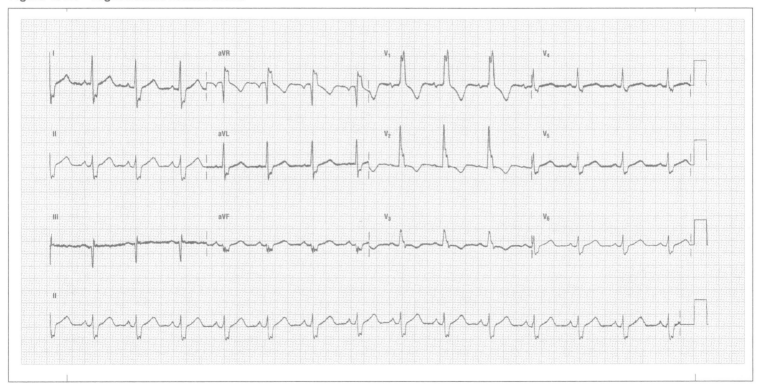

*Source*: From *12-Lead ECG: The Art of Interpretation*, courtesy of Tomas B. Garcia, MD.

## QRS complex
☒ QRS complex occurs after each P wave
☒ QRS complexes look the same in shape and size
☐ QRS complex is normal (< 0.12 sec)
☒ QRS complex is wide (≥ 0.12 sec; unless there is an incomplete RBBB where the QRS complex will be < 0.12 sec)

## QRS complex direction in $V_1$
☐ Negative
☒ Positive (if monitoring V1, a positive R wave will be visible)*
☐ Cannot determine

## Q-T interval**
☐ Normal (≤ 0.40 sec)

## QTc**
☐ Normal (men ≤ 0.44 sec, women ≤ 0.46 sec)
☐ Long or approaching the danger zone (> 0.50 sec)

## Left Bundle Branch Block

A left bundle branch block (LBBB; see Figure 16-22) is defined as a delay in the transmission of the electrical impulse from the left bundle branch to the ventricle. The delay occurs as the electrical impulse meets a block in the common left bundle, causing the electrical impulse to move slowly around the block through the surrounding muscle of the heart. While there is a delay in the transmission of the impulse down the left bundle, there is regular rapid transmission of the impulse down the right bundle. This asynchronous transmission of impulses results in depolarization of the right ventricle before the left ventricle.(Refer back to Section 6, Left Bundle Branch Block).

**Rate**
☒ Normal (60–100 beats per minute; rate depends on the underlying rhythm)
☒ Bradycardia (< 60 beats per minute)
☒ Tachycardia (> 100 beats per minute)

**Rhythm**
☒ Regular
☒ Irregular

**P waves**
☒ P wave occurs before each QRS complex
☒ P waves look the same in shape and size
❑ P waves in V1 are monophasic, < 0.12 sec in duration, < 2.5 mm (0.25 mV) in height*
❑ P waves cannot be found

**P-R interval**
☒ Normal (0.12 sec to 0.20 sec)
❑ Short (< 0.12 sec)
❑ Long (> 0.20 sec)
❑ Cannot determine

**QRS complex**
☒ QRS complex occurs after each P wave
☒ QRS complexes look the same in shape and size
❑ QRS complex is normal (< 0.12 sec)
☒ QRS complex is wide (≥ 0.12 sec)

**Figure 16-22  Left Bundle Branch Block**

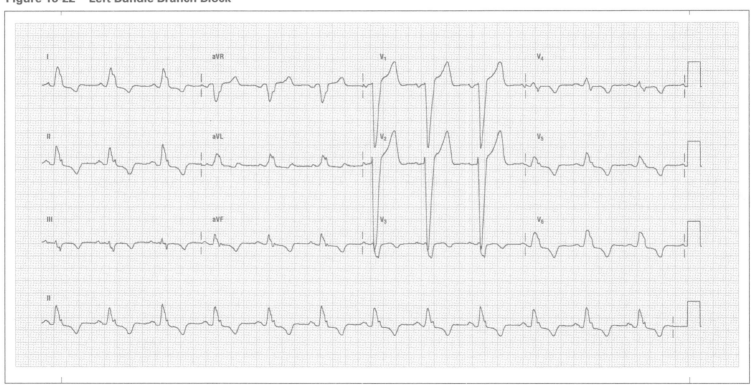

*Source*: From *12-Lead ECG: The Art of Interpretation*, courtesy of Tomas B. Garcia, MD.

## QRS complex direction in $V_1$
☒ Negative (if monitoring $V_1$, a negative R wave will be visible)
❏ Positive
❏ Cannot determine

## Q-T interval**
❏ Normal (≤ 0.40 sec)

## QTc**
❏ Normal (men ≤ 0.44 sec, women ≤ 0.46 sec)
❏ Long or approaching the danger zone (> 0.50 sec)

## Hemiblock

A hemiblock occurs when there is a block in one or more of the fascicles of the left bundle branch, that is, the anterior fascicle, the posterior fascicle, or the middle fascicle.(Refer back to Section 6, Anterior and Posterior Hemiblocks).

## Rate
☒ Normal (60–100 beats per minute; rate depends on the underlying rhythm)
☒ Bradycardia (< 60 beats per minute)
☒ Tachycardia (> 100 beats per minute)

## Rhythm
☒ Regular
☒ Irregular

### Fascicular Blocks and Mobitz Type II
A Mobitz type II second-degree heart block can occur when all of the fascicles of the heart are blocked except for one fascicle that has an intermittent block (see Figure 16-23).

**Figure 16-23    Type 11 Second-Degree Heart Block**

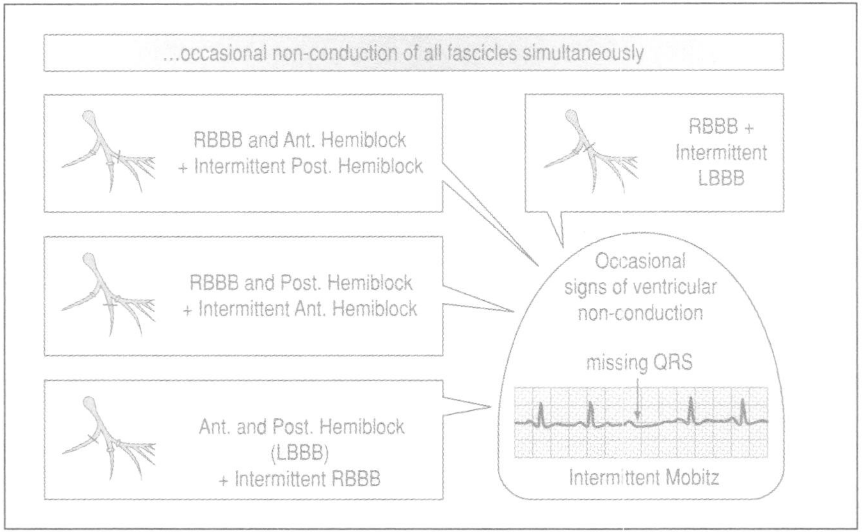

...occasional non-conduction of all fascicles simultaneously

RBBB and Ant. Hemiblock
+ Intermittent Post. Hemiblock

RBBB +
Intermittent
LBBB

RBBB and Post. Hemiblock
+ Intermittent Ant. Hemiblock

Occasional
signs of ventricular
non-conduction

missing QRS

Ant. and Post. Hemiblock
(LBBB)
+ Intermittent RBBB

Intermittent Mobitz

*Source*: Courtesy of Dale Dubin, MD & COVER Publishing Company in *Rapid Interpretation of EKGs*, 2000.

**P waves**
☒ P wave occurs before each QRS complex
☒ P waves look the same in shape and size
❑ P waves in V1 are monophasic, < 0.12 sec in duration, < 2.5 mm (0.25 mV) in height*
❑ P waves cannot be found

**P-R interval**
☒ Normal (0.12 sec to 0.20 sec)
❑ Short (< 0.12 sec)
❑ Long (> 0.20 sec)
❑ Cannot determine

**QRS complex**
☒ QRS complex occurs after each P wave
☒ QRS complexes look the same in shape and size
☒ QRS complex is normal (< 0.12 sec; QRS complex is 0.10 sec to 0.12 sec wide)
☒ QRS complex is wide (≥ 0.12 sec)

**QRS complex direction in $V_1$\***
❑ Negative
❑ Positive
❑ Cannot determine

**Q-T interval\*\***
❑ Normal (≤ 0.40 sec)

## QTc**
❑ Normal (men ≤ 0.44 sec, women ≤ 0.46 sec)
❑ Long or approaching the danger zone (> 0.50 sec)

## Pulseless Electrical Activity

Pulseless electrical activity (PEA; see Figure 16-24*) occurs when there is electrical activity of the heart but there is no mechanical contraction.

- In PEA, the patient does not have a pulse because there is no mechanical contraction of the heart.
- PEA is very deceiving because it can look like a perfusing rhythm.
- To treat PEA, it is important to identify why the electrical circuit within the heart is blocked.
- Causes of PEA include (six Hs and five Ts) (American Heart Association Handbook, 2008; American Heart Association Guidelines, 2005):
  - Hypovolemia
  - Hypoxia
  - Hydrogen ion (acidosis)
  - Hypokalemia/hyperkalemia
  - Hypoglycemia
  - Hypothermia
  - Toxins
  - Tamponade, cardiac
  - Tension pneumothorax
  - Thrombosis (coronary or pulmonary)
  - Trauma

**Figure 16-24    Pulseless Electrical Activity**

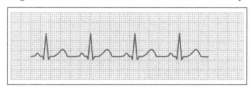

*Source*: Jackson, J. & Jackson, L. *Clinical nursing pocket guide*. Jones and Bartlett Publishers.

*Note:* *Any organized rhythm that is not associated with a pulse is interpreted as PEA.

**Rate**
☒ Normal (60–100 beats per minute)
☒ Bradycardia (< 60 beats per minute)
☒ Tachycardia (> 100 beats per minute)

**Rhythm**
☒ Regular
☒ Irregular

**P waves**
☒ P wave occurs before each QRS complex
☒ P waves look the same in shape and size
☒ P waves in V1 are monophasic, < 0.12 sec in duration, < 2.5 mm (0.25 mV) in height*
☒ P waves cannot be found

**P-R interval**
☒ Normal (0.12 sec to 0.20 sec)
☒ Short (< 0.12 sec)
☒ Long (> 0.20 sec)
☒ Cannot determine

**QRS complex**
☒ QRS complex occurs after each P wave
☒ QRS complexes look the same in shape and size
☒ QRS complex is normal (< 0.12 sec)
☒ QRS complex is wide (≥ 0.12 sec)

**QRS complex direction in $V_1$***
❑ Negative
❑ Positive
❑ Cannot determine

**Q-T interval\*\***
❑ Normal (≤ 0.40 sec)

**QTc\*\***
❑ Normal (men ≤ 0.44 sec, women ≤ 0.46 sec)
❑ Long or approaching the danger zone (> 0.50 sec)

## Asystole

Asystole (see Figure 16-25) is defined as a total absence or block of all electrical activity. The causes of asystole are the same as causes for PEA (American Heart Association Handbook, 2008; American Heart Association Guidelines, 2005).

**Figure 16-25    Asystole**

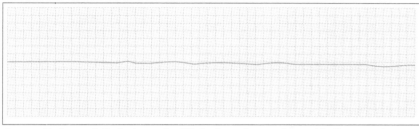

*Source*: Jackson, J. & Jackson, L. *Clinical nursing pocket guide*. Jones and Bartlett Publishers.

## Rate
❑ Normal (60–100 beats per minute)
❑ Bradycardia (< 60 beats per minute)
❑ Tachycardia (> 100 beats per minute)

## Rhythm
❑ Regular
❑ Irregular

## P waves
❑ P wave occurs before each QRS complex
❑ P waves look the same in shape and size
❑ P waves in V1 are monophasic, < 0.12 sec in duration, < 2.5 mm (0.25 mV) in height
❑ P waves cannot be found

## P-R interval
❑ Normal (0.12 sec to 0.20 sec)
❑ Short (< 0.12 sec)
❑ Long (> 0.20 sec)
❑ Cannot determine

## QRS complex
❑ QRS complex occurs after each P wave
❑ QRS complexes look the same in shape and size
❑ QRS complex is normal (< 0.12 sec)
❑ QRS complex is wide (≥ 0.12 sec)

## QRS complex direction in $V_1$
❑ Negative
❑ Positive
❑ Cannot determine

## Q-T interval
❑ Normal (≤ 0.40 sec)

## QTc
❑ Normal (men ≤ 0.44 sec, women ≤ 0.46 sec)
❑ Long or approaching the danger zone (> 0.50 sec)

---

**Asystole versus Fine Ventricular Fibrillation**

Asystole and fine ventricular fibrillation can look the same in certain leads. To assist in distinguishing one from the other, check the rhythm in a second lead.

**Tips to Assist in Differentiating Sinus Tachycardia (ST) from Supraventricular Tachycardia (SVT)**

1. Electrical impulse initiation and transmission
   ST: The electrical impulse is initiated in the sinus node.
   SVT:
   a. The electrical impulse is initiated from an increase in automaticity from one or more ectopic foci within the atria (atrial tachycardia, multifocal atrial tachycardia, and atrial fibrillation) or from within the AV junction (junctional ectopic tachycardia).
   b. The electrical impulse is initiated and sustained by a reentrant mechanism within the atria (atrial flutter).
   c. The electrical impulse is transmitted through dual pathways within the AV node (atrioventricular nodal reentrant tachycardia).
   d. The electrical impulse is transmitted through the AV node and through an accessory pathway outside of the AV node (atrioventricular bypass tachycardia).

2. P wave
   ST: P waves are upright and discernible especially in leads II, III, and aVF.
   SVT: P waves may be hidden in the QRS or the T wave. If P waves are present, they are different than the normal sinus P waves.

3. Onset of rhythm
   ST: Onset and cessation are gradual.
   SVT: Onset and cessation are sudden. Onset is often preceded by a premature ectopic beat.

4. Heart rate
   ST: Heart rate is greater than 100 but rarely exceeds 150–180 beats per minute in a resting adult (some literature sets the lower rate limit of ST in the resting adult at 120–125 beats per minute) (American Heart Association Guidelines, 2005; Dubin, 2000).
   SVT: Heart rates usually are between 150 and 250 beats per minute (Scheinman & Kaushik, 2003).

5. Miscellaneous identifiers specific for ST
   ST: Responds to carotid sinus pressure by a gradual slowing of the heart rate.
   ST: Variability in heart rate can be seen in response to respiration and to activity.

## TACHYARRHYTHMIAS

*"I think I will pump up the beat."*

Tachyarrhythmias are rhythms that are initiated in the atria, the AV junction, or the ventricles and are associated with ventricular rates greater than 150 beats per minute. These rhythms are often paroxysmal, that is, they have a sudden onset and can have a spontaneous abrupt termination. Causes of tachyarrhythmias include:

- An increase in automaticity of ectopic foci.
- An abnormal transmission of the electrical impulse through a reentrant mechanism.
- An abnormal transmission of the electrical impulse through dual pathway(s).
- An abnormal transmission of the electrical impulse through accessory pathway(s).

**Figure 16-26   Atrial Tachycardia**

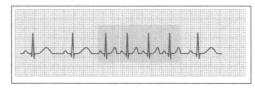

*Source*: Jackson, J. & Jackson, L. *Clinical nursing pocket guide*. Jones and Bartlett Publishers.

## Supraventricular Tachycardia

Supraventricular tachycardia (SVT) is a broad term used to describe tachyarrhythmias that occur above the ventricle, that is, in the atria and in or around the AV junction (the AV junction includes the AV node and the His bundle). The SVT arrhythmias include:

- Atrial tachycardia
- Multifocal atrial tachycardia
- Atrial flutter
- Atrial fibrillation
- Junctional ectopic tachycardia
- Atrioventricular nodal reentrant tachycardia (AVNRT)
- Atrioventricular bypass tachycardia (AVBT)

### Atrial Tachycardia

Atrial tachycardia (see Figure 16-26) is a supraventricular tachycardia that occurs when there is an increase in automaticity of a single ectopic focus within the atria that causes electrical impulses to be initiated and transmitted to the ventricles at a rate of 150–250 beats per minute.

- Patients should be screened for "tachycardia induced cardiomyopathy" that can occur with frequent bouts of this arrhythmia (Ganz, 2003, p. 172).
- Although it is rare, digitalis toxicity is the "most common cause "of this arrhythmia (Wagner & Wang, 2008a, p. 293).

### Rate
❑ Normal (60–100 beats per minute)
❑ Bradycardia (< 60 beats per minute)
☒ Tachycardia (> 100 beats per minute; rate is often 150–250 beats per minute)

**Rhythm**
☒ Regular
❑ Irregular

**P waves**
☒ P wave occurs before each QRS complex (P waves may be hidden in the preceding T wave)
☒ P waves look the same in shape and size (but the morphology of the P wave that is associated with the arrhythmia differs from the normal sinus P wave)
❑ P waves in $V_1$ are monophasic, < 0.12 sec in duration, < 2.5 mm (0.25 mV) in height*
❑ P waves cannot be found

**P-R interval**
☒ Normal (0.12 sec to 0.20 sec; P-R interval may be different than the P-R interval associated with the normal sinus beat; in digitalis toxicity the P-R interval may be lengthened)
❑ Short (< 0.12 sec)
❑ Long (> 0.20 sec)
❑ Cannot determine

**QRS complex**
☒ QRS complex occurs after each P wave (may have a variable AV block)
☒ QRS complexes look the same in shape and size
☒ QRS complex is normal (< 0.12 sec)
❑ QRS complex is wide (≥ 0.12 sec)

**QRS complex direction in $V_1$***
❑ Negative
❑ Positive
❑ Cannot determine

**Q-T interval\*\***
❑ Normal (≤ 0.40 sec)

**QTc\*\***
❑ Normal (men ≤ 0.44 sec, women ≤ 0.46 sec)
❑ Long or approaching the danger zone (> 0.50 sec)

### *Multifocal Atrial Tachycardia*

Multifocal atrial tachycardia (MAT; see Figure 16-27), also called "chaotic atrial tachycardia" (Wagner & Wang, 2008a, p. 294), is a supraventricular tachycardia that occurs when there is an increase in automaticity of multiple ectopic foci within the atria that causes electrical impulses to be initiated and transmitted to the ventricles at a rate greater than 100–120 beats per minute. MAT is often a side effect of conditions such as chronic obstructive pulmonary disease (McCord & Borzak, 1698), diabetes, cardiorespiratory illnesses, and administration of proarrhythmic medications (Conover, 2003).

**Figure 16-27    Multifocal Atrial Tachycardia**

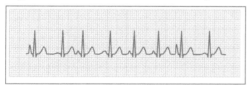

*Source*: Jackson, J. & Jackson, L. *Clinical nursing pocket guide*. Jones and Bartlett Publishers.

## Rate
☐ Normal (60–100 beats per minute)
☐ Bradycardia (< 60 beats per minute)
☒ Tachycardia (> 100 beats per minute; rates are often > 100–120 beats per minute)

## Rhythm
☐ Regular
☒ Irregular

## P waves
☒ P wave occurs before each QRS complex (the morphology of the P wave differs from the morphology of the normal sinus P wave; in MAT there are at least three different P wave morphologies)
☐ P waves look the same in shape and size
☐ P waves in V1 are monophasic, < 0.12 sec in duration, < 2.5 mm (0.25 mV) in height*
☐ P waves cannot be found

## P-R interval
☒ Normal (0.12 sec to 0.20 sec; P-R interval may vary)
☐ Short (< 0.12 sec)
☐ Long (> 0.20 sec)
☐ Cannot determine

## QRS complex
☒ QRS complex occurs after each P wave
☒ QRS complexes look the same in shape and size
☒ QRS complex is normal (< 0.12 sec)
☐ QRS complex is wide (≥ 0.12 sec)

## QRS complex direction in $V_1$*
❑ Negative
❑ Positive
❑ Cannot determine

## Q-T interval**
❑ Normal (≤ 0.40 sec)

## QTc**
❑ Normal (men ≤ 0.44 sec, women ≤ 0.46 sec)
❑ Long or approaching the danger zone (> 0.50 sec)

### *Atrial Flutter*

Atrial flutter (see Figure 16-28) is a supraventricular tachycardia that occurs when a premature ectopic foci within the atria, usually within the right atria, initiates a reentrant mechanism that results in a continual circle of electrical activity within the atria. This reentrant mechanism produces P waves, referred to as flutter waves or F waves, at rates between 220 and 350 beats per minute (usually around 300 beats per minute), which are best seen in leads II, III, and $aV_F$ (Wagner, 2008). There will usually be a block of one-half of the F waves within the AV node (if the AV node is functioning normally) to protect the ventricles from receiving excessive electrical impulses. For example: An atrial rate of 300 will result in a ventricular rate of 150 because of the AV node "protection."

**Figure 16-28   Atrial Flutter**

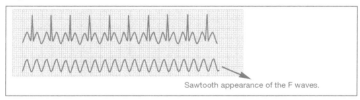

Sawtooth appearance of the F waves.

*Source*: Jackson, J. & Jackson, L. *Clinical nursing pocket guide.*
Jones and Bartlett Publishers.

- The F waves often have a sawtooth appearance.
- Atrial flutter can be seen after cardiac surgery, after myocardial infarction, with mitral or tricuspid valve disease, or with other congenital abnormalities (Scheinman & Kaushik, 2003).

> Tip: Look for flutter waves in any narrow complex tachycardia with a rate of 150 bpm.

- Dubin (2000) suggests inverting the rhythm strip to assist in the identification of atrial flutter.
- There are two types of atrial flutter: typical and atypical (Scheinman & Kaushik, 2003).
  - Typical atrial flutter is the most common type and is associated with:
    - Negative F waves in II, III, and $aV_F$, and positive F waves in V1 (counterclockwise flutter) or positive F waves in II, III, and $aV_F$, and negative F waves in V1 (clockwise flutter)
    - An F wave rate that is regular and rapid, usually around 300 beats per minute.
- Atypical atrial flutter is associated with:
  - Postive or negative F waves in II, III, and $aV_F$
  - An F wave rate that is irregular and rapid, usually around 350 beats per minute.
  - Atrial fibrillation. Atypical atrial flutter can precede the onset of atrial fibrillation.

## Rate
- ❑ Normal (60–100 beats per minute)
- ❑ Bradycardia (< 60 beats per minute)
- ☒ Tachycardia (> 100 beats per minute; although the atrial rate is usually around 300 beats per minute the ventricular rate is 150–170 beats per minute because of AV node protection).

## Rhythm
- ☒ Regular (usually regular but may vary depending on the variability of the AV conduction)
- ❑ Irregular

**P waves**
- ❏ P wave occurs before each QRS complex
- ❏ P waves look the same in shape and size
- ❏ P waves in $V_1$ are monophasic, < 0.12 sec in duration, < 2.5 mm (0.25 mV) in height
- ☒ P waves cannot be found (P waves are replaced by flutter or F waves. F waves can have a sawtooth pattern, can be negative or positive depending on the lead being used for monitoring, and can be hidden in the QRS or the T wave.

**P-R interval**
- ❏ Normal (0.12 sec to 0.20 sec)
- ❏ Short (< 0.12 sec)
- ❏ Long (> 0.20 sec)
- ☒ Cannot determine

**QRS complex**
- ❏ QRS complex occurs after each P wave
- ☒ QRS complexes look the same in shape and size
- ☒ QRS complex is normal (< 0.12 sec)
- ❏ QRS complex is wide (≥ 0.12 sec)

**QRS complex direction in $V_1$***
- ❏ Negative
- ❏ Positive
- ❏ Cannot determine

**Q-T interval****
- ❏ Normal (≤ 0.40 sec)

QTc**
❏ Normal (men ≤ 0.44 sec, women ≤ 0.46 sec)
❏ Long or approaching the danger zone (> 0.50 sec)

## *Atrial Fibrillation*

Atrial fibrillation (see Figure 16-29) is a supraventricular tachyarrhythmia that occurs when electrical impulses throughout the left and right atria are initiated in an erratic and rapid fashion, producing P waves (although the P waves usually cannot be seen on the EKG) at rates of 350–450 beats per minute that vary in shape, size, and amplitude. This erratic and rapid initiation of electrical impulses is often initiated by a premature atrial beat(s) and causes the atria to quiver, increasing the risk of thrombus formation and predisposing the patient to stroke, myocardial infarction, hemodynamic compromise, and more. The ventricular response to these electrical impulses is irregular and can be fast or slow depending on the number of atrial electrical impulses that are conducted through the AV node.

**Figure 16-29   Atrial Fibrillation**

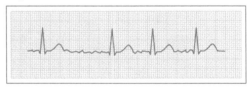

*Source*: Jackson, J. & Jackson, L. *Clinical nursing pocket guide*. Jones and Bartlett Publishers.

- After a myocardial infarction, 10-15% of patients have atrial fibrillation (Hebbar & Hueston, 2002).
- Atrial fibrillation is the most common complication after cardiac surgery (Kern, McRae, & Funk, 2007). It has been reported that after open heart surgery, 30% of patients can have atrial fibrillation (Kramer, Ide, & Drew, 1999), and 70% of the cases are seen on postoperative days two to four (Kern, et al., 2007).
- After a valve replacement, 60% of patients can have atrial fibrillation (Kramer, et al., 1999).
- A change in the structure or the function of the atria can increase the risk of atrial fibrillation (Nattel, Burstein, & Dobrev, 2008).
- Symptoms often associated with atrial fibrillation are shortness of breath, palpitations, chest pain, fatigue (Ezekowitz, 2007), light-headedness, dizziness, and anxiety; however, some patients do not experience any symptoms (Kern, et al., 2007).
- Atrial fibrillation is the most common sustained cardiac rhythm disorder, and the risk of atrial fibrillation increases with age. It is estimated that 15.9 million people will have atrial fibrillation by 2050 (Lip & Tse, 2007).
- The QT/QT c is very difficult to measure in patients with atrial fibrillation because the R-R interval is so irregular. To determine if the QT is prolonged in this rhythm, use a long strip and assess if the interval from the "R wave to T peak is more than 50% of the RR interval." If it is greater than 50% of the R-R interval, the QT (c ) would be considered to be in the danger zone (Sommargren & Drew, 2007, p. 288). (Refer back to Section 9 to review another calculation that can be used for patients in atrial fibrillation).
- If atrial epicardial pacing wires are left in place after cardiac surgery and the clinician is having difficulty in determining the type of rhythm on the EKG monitor, an atrial electrogram can be obtained if hospital policy allows.

## Rate
- ❏ Normal (60–100 beats per minute)
- ❏ Bradycardia (< 60 beats per minute)
- ☒ Tachycardia (> 100 beats per minute; although the atrial rate is 350–450 beats per minute the ventricular rate is 100–160 beats per minute because of AV node protection)

## Rhythm
☐ Regular
☒ Irregular

## P waves
☐ P wave occurs before each QRS complex
☐ P waves look the same in shape and size
☐ P waves in $V_1$ are monophasic, < 0.12 sec in duration, < 2.5 mm (0.25 mV) in height
☒ P waves cannot be found

## P-R interval
☐ Normal (0.12 sec to 0.20 sec)
☐ Short (< 0.12 sec)
☐ Long (> 0.20 sec)
☒ Cannot determine

## QRS complex
☐ QRS complex occurs after each P wave
☒ QRS complexes look the same in shape and size
☒ QRS complex is normal (< 0.12 sec)
☐ QRS complex is wide (≥ 0.12 sec)

## QRS complex direction in $V_1$*
☐ Negative
☐ Positive
☐ Cannot determine

**Q-T interval\*\***
❑ Normal (≤ 0.40 sec)

**QTc\*\***
❑ Normal (men ≤ 0.44 sec, women ≤ 0.46 sec)
❑ Long or approaching the danger zone (> 0.50 sec)

### *Junctional Ectopic Tachycardia*

Junctional ectopic tachycardia (JET; see Figure 16-30) is a rare supraventricular tachycardia that occurs primarily in infants and children and is associated with significant mortality (Zeigler & Gillette, 2001). The primary causes of JET include congenital abnormalities and postcardiac surgery (Andreasen, Johnsen, & Ravn, 2008; Zeigler & Gillette, 2001). JET is triggered by an increase in automaticity of an ectopic foci around the AV junction (AV node and the bundle of His) due to irritation, trauma, inflammation, or a dopamine infusion (Horenstein, 2008).

**Figure 16-30  Junctional Ectopic Tachycardia**

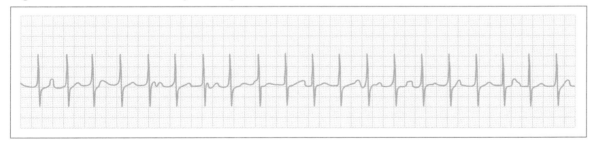

## Rate
- ❑ Normal (60–100 beats per minute)
- ❑ Bradycardia (< 60 beats per minute)
- ☒ Tachycardia (> 100 beats per minute; ventricular rates can vary between 110 and 250 beats per minute, but they can be as high as 370 beats per minute)

## Rhythm
- ☒ Regular (slight variation of the heart rate may be seen)
- ❑ Irregular

## P waves
- ❑ P wave occurs before each QRS complex
- ❑ P waves look the same in shape and size
- ❑ P waves in V1 are monophasic, < 0.12 sec in duration, < 2.5 mm (0.25 mV) in height*
- ☒ P waves cannot be found (P waves are often hidden in the QRS or T wave and are disassociated from the QRS complex)

## P-R interval
- ❑ Normal (0.12 sec to 0.20 sec)
- ❑ Short (< 0.12 sec)
- ❑ Long (> 0.20 sec)
- ☒ Cannot determine

## QRS complex
- ❑ QRS complex occurs after each P wave
- ☒ QRS complexes look the same in shape and size
- ☒ QRS complex is normal (< 0.12 sec)
- ❑ QRS complex is wide (≥ 0.12 sec)

**QRS complex direction in $V_1$***
❑ Negative
❑ Positive
❑ Cannot determine

**Q-T interval****
❑ Normal (≤ 0.40 sec)

**QTc***
❑ Normal (men ≤ 0.44 sec, women ≤ 0.46 sec)
❑ Long or approaching the danger zone (> 0.50 sec)

> *Note:* In normal conditions when an electrical impulse is initiated, the impulse travels down the fast pathway through the AV node.

> *Note:* The retrograde movement of the electrical impulse from the ventricle to the atria can result in an inverse P wave immediately before the QRS, a P wave immediately after the QRS, or no P waves at all (Gilbert & Wagner, 2008a.)

### Atrioventricular Nodal Reentrant Tachycardia

Atrioventricular nodal reentrant tachycardia (AVNRT; see Figure 16-31) is the most common type of supraventricular tachycardia (Katritis & Camm, 2006). One-half of patients with symptomatic paroxysmal supraventricular tachycardia are in AVNRT (Conover, 2003).

This reentrant tachycardia occurs because of the presence of dual pathways within the AV node. These pathways are referred to as the fast pathway and the slow pathway, and each pathway has a different conduction velocity and a different refractory period (Jacobson, 2007).

In typical AVNRT a premature atrial beat is initiated and is transmitted down the slow pathway in an antegrade fashion to the ventricles because the fast pathway has not completely repolarized from the previous electrical impulse. The impulse then travels back up to the atria in a retrograde fashion through the now repolarized fast pathway. This retrograde/antegrade sequence will continue, thereby creating a reentrant tachycardia as the electrical impulse travels down one pathway and back up the other in a rapid successive fashion (Heidbuchel & Jackman, 2004; see Figure 16-32). (Antegrade and retrograde conduction are defined in Section 6 under the AV Node heading.)

**Figure 16-31    Atrioventricular Nodal Reentrant Tachycardia (AVNRT)**

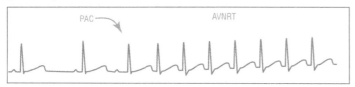

*Source*: Rosenthal, L. S. *Dx/Rx: Arrhythmia.* © 2008 Jones and Bartlett Publishers.

**Figure 16-32    Typical AVNRT Slow-Fast**

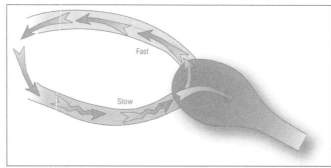

*Source*: Rosenthal, L. S. *Dx/Rx: Arrhythmia.* © 2008 Jones and Bartlett Publishers.

- In typical AVNRT the electrical impulse travels down the slow pathway and up the fast pathway (slow–fast; Heidbuchel & Jackman, 2004).
- In atypical AVNRT the electrical impulse travels down the fast pathway and up the slow pathway (fast–slow) or down the slow pathway and up the slow pathway (slow–slow).
  - AVNRT has an abrupt onset.
  - Two-thirds of patients have no visible P waves (Gilbert & Wagner, 2008a).
  - One-third of patients have a P wave after the QRS (Gilbert & Wagner, 2008a).
  - Very few patients have P waves before the QRS (Gilbert & Wagner, 2008a).
  - If P waves are seen, they will be inverted and will be part of the QRS complex. This can distort the morphology of the QRS complex by creating a "'pseudo-S-wave' in leads II, III, $aV_F$ or 'pseudo-R-wave' in lead $V_1$" (Gilbert & Wagner, 2008a, p. 336).

## Rate
❑ Normal (60–100 beats per minute)
❑ Bradycardia (< 60 beats per minute)
☒ Tachycardia (> 100 beats per minute; rate of 140-200 beats per minute, but it can be faster)

## Rhythm
☒ Regular
❑ Irregular

## P waves
❑ P wave occurs before each QRS complex
❑ P waves look the same in shape and size
❑ P waves in V1 are monophasic, < 0.12 sec in duration, < 2.5 mm (0.25 mV) in height
☒ P waves cannot be found (the majority of patients have no visible P wave)

## P-R interval
❑ Normal (0.12 sec to 0.20 sec)
❑ Short (< 0.12 sec)
❑ Long (> 0.20 sec)
☒ Cannot determine

## QRS complex
❑ QRS complex occurs after each P wave
☒ QRS complexes look the same in shape and size (if an inverted P wave is present the QRS morphology could be distorted)
☒ QRS complex is normal (< 0.12 sec)
❑ QRS complex is wide (≥ 0.12 sec)

**QRS complex direction in V$_1$***
- ❏ Negative
- ❏ Positive
- ❏ Cannot determine

**Q-T interval****
- ❏ Normal (≤ 0.40 sec)

**QTc****
- ❏ Normal (men ≤ 0.44 sec, women ≤ 0.46 sec)
- ❏ Long or approaching the danger zone (> 0.50 sec)

### *Atrioventricular Bypass Tachycardia*

Atrioventricular bypass tachycardia (AVBT; see Figure 16-33) is also called atrioventricular reciprocating tachycardia (AVRT), circus movement tachycardia (CMT) with an accessory pathway, orthodromic AV-bypass tachycardia, or antidromic AV-bypass tachycardia. It is considered to be a supraventricular tachycardia and occurs with an abrupt onset when a premature atrial beat is initiated and transmitted in an orthodromic or antidromic fashion (Jacobson, 2007) through two pathways: the AV node and an accessory pathway outside of the AV node.

In orthodromic AVBT, which occurs more frequently than antidromic, the electrical impulse travels down the AV node and the accessory pathway, then it proceeds up the accessory pathway and back down the AV node in a rapid, successive, circus-type fashion. Wolff-Parkinson-White (WPW) syndrome is the most common type of orthodromic AV-bypass tachycardia. In WPW the accessory pathway has been called the Kent bundle. (WPW is discussed in Section 7 under the Accessory Pathways heading.)

In antidromic AVBT the electrical impulse travels up the AV node, down the accessory pathway, and then back up the AV node in a rapid, successive, circus-type fashion.

**Rate**
- ❏ Normal (60–100 beats per minute)

**Figure 16-33    Atrioventricular Bypass Tachycardia (AVBT)**

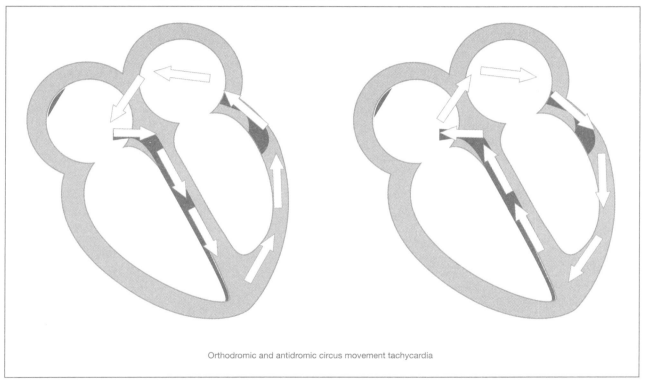

Orthodromic and antidromic circus movement tachycardia

*Source*: From AACN Advanced Critical Care, Jacobson, Carol/Funk, Marjorie, 18 (3): Figure 14: Orthodromic and antidromic. *Narrow QRS Complex Tachycardias*, Copyright 2007.

❏ Bradycardia (< 60 beats per minute)
☒ Tachycardia (> 100 beats per minute; rate is 150–250 beats per minute, often > 200)

> *Note:* In WPW a P wave can be present with slower heart rates and the P-R interval will usually be short).

**Rhythm**
☒ Regular (may be slightly irregular)
❏ Irregular

**P waves**
❏ P wave occurs before each QRS complex
❏ P waves look the same in shape and size
❏ P waves in V1 are monophasic, < 0.12 sec in duration, < 2.5 mm (0.25 mV) in height
☒ P waves cannot be found (P waves can be hidden in the ST segment or T waves )

**P-R interval**
❏ Normal (0.12 sec to 0.20 sec)
❏ Short (< 0.12 sec)
❏ Long (> 0.20 sec)
☒ Cannot determine

**QRS complex**
❏ QRS complex occurs after each P wave
☒ QRS complexes look the same in shape and size
☒ QRS complex is normal (< 0.12 sec)
☒ QRS complex is wide (≥ 0.12 sec; in WPW the QRS can be widened and can have a delta wave)

**QRS complex direction in V₁***
❑ Negative
❑ Positive
❑ Cannot determine

**Q-T interval****
❑ Normal (≤ 0.40 sec)

**QTc****
❑ Normal (men ≤ 0.44 sec, women ≤ 0.46 sec)
❑ Long or approaching the danger zone (> 0.50 sec)

## Ventricular Tachycardia

Ventricular tachycardia (VT; see Figure 16-34), also referred to as ventricular flutter or monomorphic ventricular tachycardia, occurs when there is an increase in automaticity of a single ectopic focus within the ventricle that triggers a reentrant cycle of electrical activity within the ventricle (Gilbert & Wagner, 2008b) at a rate greater than 100 beats per minute. Ventricular tachycardia is paroxysmal, regular, and orderly and can deteriorate into ventricular fibrillation if left untreated (Gilbert & Wagner, 2008b). Because the electrical impulse occurs in the ventricle, the QRS complex is wide and bizarre.

**Figure 16-34   Ventricular Tachycardia**

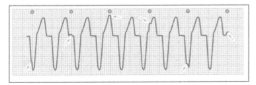

*Source*: Jackson, J. & Jackson, L. *Clinical nursing pocket guide*. Jones and Bartlett Publishers.

## Rate
☐ Normal (60–100 beats per minute)
☐ Bradycardia (< 60 beats per minute)
☒ Tachycardia (> 100 beats per minute; rates can vary between 100 and 250 beats per minute)

## Rhythm
☒ Regular
☐ Irregular

## P waves
☐ P wave occurs before each QRS complex
☐ P waves look the same in shape and size
☐ P waves in V1 are monophasic, < 0.12 sec in duration, < 2.5 mm (0.25 mV) in height
☒ P waves cannot be found (P waves are hidden within the QRS complex)

## P-R interval
☐ Normal (0.12 sec to 0.20 sec)
☐ Short (< 0.12 sec)
☐ Long (> 0.20 sec)
☒ Cannot determine

## QRS complex
☐ QRS complex occurs after each P wave
☒ QRS complexes look the same in shape and size
☐ QRS complex is normal (< 0.12 sec)
☒ QRS complex is wide (≥ 0.12 sec; QRS complex is wide and bizarre)

> *Note:* The sinus node will continue to attempt to pace the heart during ventricular tachycardia but the P-waves will not be seen or may be buried within the QRS complex and can be marched out.

**QRS complex direction in $V_1$*
- ❑ Negative
- ❑ Positive
- ☒ Cannot determine

**Q-T interval**
- ❑ Normal ($\leq$ 0.40 sec)
- ☒ Cannot determine

**QTc**
- ❑ Normal (men $\leq$ 0.44 sec, women $\leq$ 0.46 sec)
- ❑ Long or approaching the danger zone (> 0.50 sec)
- ☒ Cannot determine

- After an acute myocardial infarction, 60 % of patients can have ventricular tachycardia (Hebbar & Hueston, 2002).
- Researchers have found that some patients have a genetic "glitch" in their electrical conduction system that can cause an abnormal heart rhythm. RyR2 is a gene that has been found to cause a genetic glitch that can lead to catecholaminergic polymorphic ventricular tachycardia (Mayo Clinic, 2005, para. 10; Taggart, et al., 2007).
- Brugada syndrome can lead to rapid polymorphic ventricular tachycardia or ventricular fibrillation (Scheinman & Kaushik, 2003).
- Idiopathic hypertrophic cardiomyopathy is "the most common genetic cardiovascular disease transmitted as an autosomal dominant trait" (Poliac, Barron, & Maron, 2006, p. 183). It can lead to malignant ventricular tachycardia (Hebbar & Hueston, 2002) and atrial fibrillation.
- Ventricular tachycardia greater than 30 sec is a medical emergency (Hebbar & Hueston, 2002).
- Three or more consecutive premature ventricular beats is defined as ventricular tachycardia.
- Supraventricular tachycardia (SVT) with aberrancy can look like ventricular tachycardia.

## Ventricular Fibrillation

Ventricular fibrillation (see Figure 16-35) occurs when there is an increase in automaticity of multiple ectopic foci within the ventricle that triggers a reentrant cycle of turbulent and irregular electrical activity within the ventricle (Gilbert & Wagner, 2008b) at rates of 350–450 beats per minute (Dubin, 2000). Ventricular fibrillation requires immediate treatment because the rhythm cannot produce a pulse or a blood pressure.

**Figure 16-35    Ventricular Fibrillation**

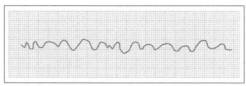

*Source*: Jackson, J. & Jackson, L. *Clinical nursing pocket guide*. Jones and Bartlett Publishers.

### Rate
- ❑ Normal (60–100 beats per minute)
- ❑ Bradycardia (< 60 beats per minute)
- ☒ Tachycardia (> 100 beats per minute; although rates have been reported to be 350–450 beats per minute, it is impossible to visually determine the rate when analyzing the strip)

### Rhythm
- ❑ Regular
- ☒ Irregular

## P waves

❏ P wave occurs before each QRS complex
❏ P waves look the same in shape and size
❏ P waves in $V_1$ are monophasic, < 0.12 sec in duration, < 2.5 mm (0.25 mV) in height
☒ P waves cannot be found

## P-R interval

❏ Normal (0.12 sec to 0.20 sec)
❏ Short (< 0.12 sec)
❏ Long (> 0.20 sec)
☒ Cannot determine

## QRS complex

❏ QRS complex occurs after each P wave
❏ QRS complexes look the same in shape and size
❏ QRS complex is normal (< 0.12 sec)
❏ QRS complex is wide (≥ 0.12 sec)
☒ No QRS complex (the ventricle is just 'quivering').

## QRS complex direction in $V_1$

❏ Negative
❏ Positive
☒ Cannot determine

## Q-T interval

❏ Normal (≤ 0.40 sec)
☒ Cannot determine

---

**SVT with Aberrant Conduction versus VT**

Some tips to assist in differentiating SVT with aberrant conduction from VT are as follows (Note: Most wide complex tachyarrhythmias are ventricular in origin):

• QRS complex
  ▪ SVT: QRS complex is < than 0.12 sec.
  ▪ VT: QRS complex is ≥ to 0.12 sec and its appearance can be wide and bizarre.
• P waves
  ▪ SVT: If P waves are present, they are synchronous with the QRS complex (although they may be hidden).
  ▪ VT: P waves and QRS complex are asynchronous from one another.
• T wave
  ▪ SVT: The deflection of the T-wave is in the same direction as the QRS complex.
  ▪ VT: The deflection of the T-wave is opposite in direction from the QRS complex.

## QTc
☐ Normal (men ≤ 0.44 sec, women ≤ 0.46 sec)
☐ Long or approaching the danger zone (> 0.50 sec)
☒ Cannot determine

### Torsades de Pointes

Torsades de pointes (see Figure 16-36) is a French term that means "twistings of the points" (Gilbert & Wagner, 2008b, p. 363). It is a polymorphic form of ventricular tachycardia that is preceded by prolongation of the QT/QTc interval (Pugh, 2000) along with a premature ventricular beat occurring on or around the T wave. Because the rhythm is often preceded by a premature ventricular beat that occurs on or around the T wave, it is referred to as the R-on-T phenomenon. Torsades de pointes often appears as an "undulating sinusoidal rhythm" in which the axis of the ventricular complex "changes from positive to negative and back in a haphazard fashion" (Garcia & Holtz, 2001, p. 530).

**Figure 16-36    Torsades de Pointes**

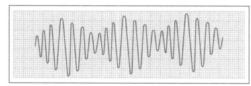

*Source*: Jackson, J. & Jackson, L. *Clinical nursing pocket guide*. Jones and Bartlett Publishers.

**Rate**
- ❑ Normal (60–100 beats per minute)
- ❑ Bradycardia (< 60 beats per minute)
- ☒ Tachycardia (> 100 beats per minute; rates vary from 180 to 250 beats per minute)

**Rhythm**
- ❑ Regular
- ☒ Irregular

**P waves**
- ❑ P wave occurs before each QRS complex
- ❑ P waves look the same in shape and size
- ❑ P waves in V1 are monophasic, < 0.12 sec in duration, < 2.5 mm (0.25 mV) in height
- ☒ P waves cannot be found

**P-R interval**
- ❑ Normal (0.12 sec to 0.20 sec)
- ❑ Short (< 0.12 sec)
- ❑ Long (> 0.20 sec)
- ☒ Cannot determine

**QRS complex**
- ❑ QRS complex occurs after each P wave
- ❑ QRS complexes look the same in shape and size
- ❑ QRS complex is normal (< 0.12 sec)
- ❑ QRS complex is wide (≥ 0.12 sec)
- ☒ No QRS complex

## QRS complex direction in V$_1$
❏ Negative
❏ Positive
☒ Cannot determine

## Q-T interval
❏ Normal ($\leq$ 0.40 sec)
☒ Cannot determine

## QTc
❏ Normal (men $\leq$ 0.44 sec, women $\leq$ 0.46 sec)
❏ Long or approaching the danger zone (> 0.50 sec)
☒ Cannot determine

Early warning signs of torsades de pointes are QTc interval > 0.50 sec, polymorphic ventricular premature beats or couplets, large U waves, nonsustained polymorphic ventricular tachycardia, a slowing heart rate, compensatory pauses, and/or T wave alternans (visible differences in the amplitude of the T wave with every other beat) (Sommargren & Drew, 2007).

### Pacemakers and rhythm strips:

A cardiac pacemaker is an electronic device that is designed to initiate and transmit electrical energy to the heart to control the patient's heart rate and rhythm when the natural pacemaker is unable to do so. Pacing can be accomplished through a permanent implantable system or through temporary systems such as a transcutaneous pacing system (Figure 16-36a) or epicardial pacing wires that are sutured to the outside surface of the ventricular wall during cardiac surgery (refer back to Section 6, Purkinje Fibers). The rhythm strip can assist in identifying if the pacemaker is functioning properly, that is, is the pacemaker capturing and sensing appropriately.

- Capture: Pacemaker capture occurs when the pacemaker successfully initiates and transmits electrical energy to the atrium, the ventricle, or both resulting in contraction of the heart (see Figure 16-37).
- Noncapture: Pacemaker noncapture occurs when the pacemaker is unsuccessful in its delivery of the electrical energy (see Figure 16-38). Failure to capture can be caused by but is not limited to the following (Lloyd & Hayes, 2000):

**Figure 16-36a   Transcutaneous pacing system**

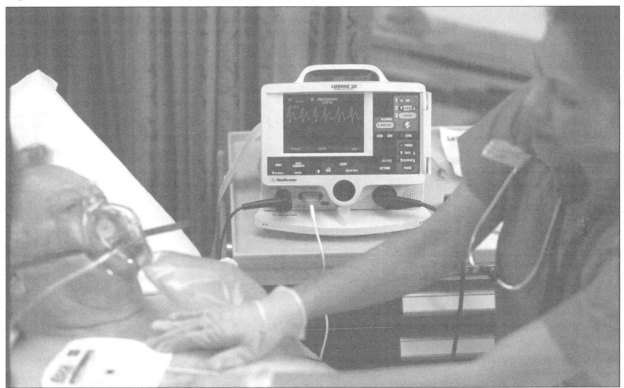

*Source*: Courtesy of Physio-Control, Inc.

**Figure 16-37   Appropriately capturing and sensing**

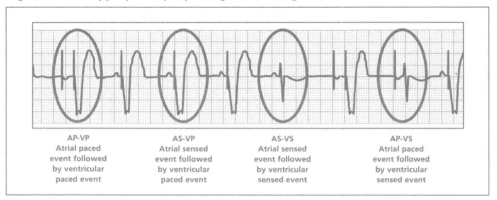

| AP-VP | AS-VP | AS-VS | AP-VS |
|---|---|---|---|
| Atrial paced event followed by ventricular paced event | Atrial sensed event followed by ventricular paced event | Atrial sensed event followed by ventricular sensed event | Atrial paced event followed by ventricular sensed event |

*Source*: Courtesy of St. Jude Medical S. C., Inc.

- Inadequate programming, that is, electrical voltage is too low
- Lead dislodgement, fracture, or perforation
- Impending battery depletion
- Poor connections
- Circuit failure
- Functional noncapture
- Sense: Pacemaker sensing occurs when the pacemaker appropriately senses the electrical activity occurring within the atrium, the ventricle, or both and only transmits electrical energy when needed (see Figure 16-37).
- Undersense: Pacemaker undersensing occurs when the pacemaker is unable to sense the electrical activity occurring within the heart and inappropriately transmits electrical energy to the heart when it is not needed (see Figure 16-39).

**Figure 16-38   Loss of capture**

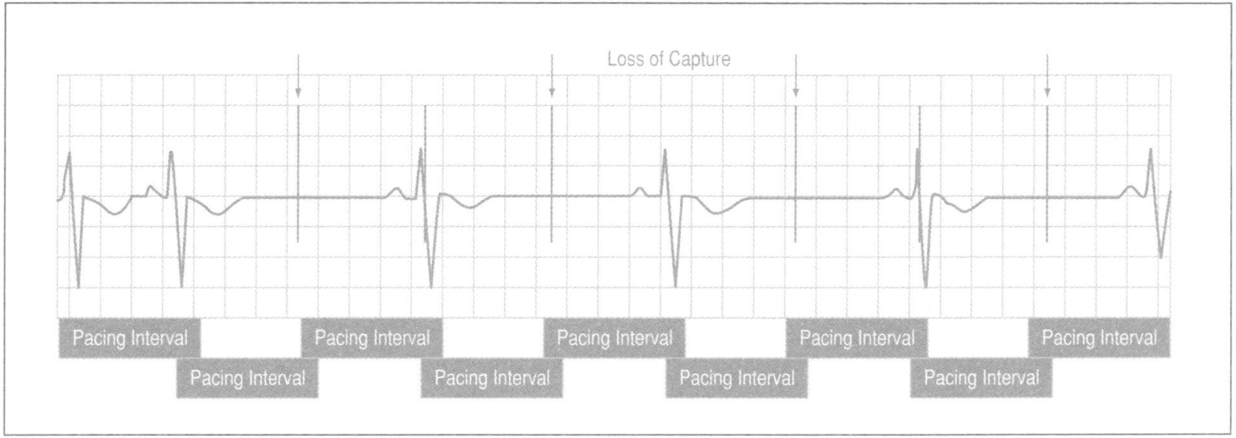

Loss of Capture

Pacing Interval

*Source*: Courtesy of St. Jude Medical S. C., Inc.

Undersensing can be caused by but is not limited to the following (Lloyd & Hayes, 2000):

- Lead dislodgement or poor lead positioning
- Application of a magnet to the pacemaker
- Electromagnetic interference
- Battery depletion

**Figure 16-39  Pacemaker undersensing**

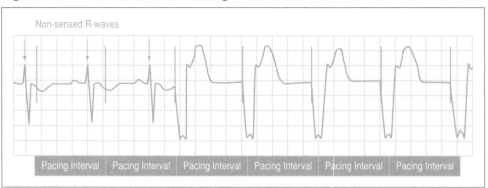

*Source*: Courtesy of St. Jude Medical S. C., Inc.

- ■ Circuit failure
- ■ Change in morphology of the patient's intrinsic EKG complexes (different from those measured at implantation)
- ■ Poor connections
- • Oversense: Pacemaker oversensing occurs when the pacemaker senses too much electrical activity occurring within the heart, including electrical interference, and fails to transmit electrical energy to the heart when it is needed (see Figure 16-40).

**Figure 16-40    Pacemaker oversensing**

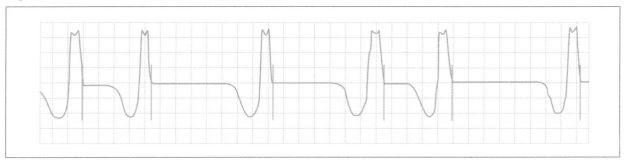

*Source*: Courtesy of St. Jude Medical S. C., Inc.

> *Note:* Permanent pacemakers have many other functions that will not be covered in this handbook.

# References

ACC/AHA/HRS. (2006). 2006 key data elements and definitions for electrophysiological studies and procedures: A report of the American College of Cardiology/American Heart Association task force on clinical data standards (ACC/AHA/HRS Writing committee to develop data standards on electrophysiology). *Circulation, 114,* 2534–2570. Retrieved June 4, 2008, from http://circ.ahajournals.org/cgi/reprint/114/23/2534

ACC/AHA/HRS. (2008). 2008 guidelines for device-based therapy of cardiac rhythm abnormalities. *Journal of American College of Cardiology, 51,* 1–62. Retrieved June 12, 2008, from http://content.onlinejacc.org/cgi/content/full/51/21/e1#TBL1

ACC Clinical Data Standards. (2001). American College of Cardiology key data elements and definitions for measuring the clinical management and outcomes of patients with acute coronary syndrome. *Journal of the American College of Cardiology, 38*(7), 2114–2130. Retrieved June 2, 2008, from http://www.acc.org/qualityandscience/clinical/data_standards/ACS/pdf/ACS_clinicaldata.pdf

Achar, S. A., Kundu, S., & Norcross, W. A. (2005). Diagnosis of acute coronary syndrome. *American Family Physician, 72*(1), 119–126. Retrieved March 28, 2008, from ProQuest Nursing & Allied Health Source.

Adams, M. G., & Pelter, M. M. (2005). Bedside monitoring of spinal cord injuries. *American Journal of Critical Care, 14*(1), 85–86.

Adams-Hamoda, M. G., Caldwell, M. A., Stotts, N. A., & Drew, B. J. (2003). Factors to consider when analyzing 12-lead electrocardiograms for evidence of acute myocardial ischemia. *American Journal of Critical Care, 12*(1), 9–16. Retrieved May 13, 2008, from http://ajcc.aacnjournals.org/cgi/content/full/12/1/9

Al-Khatib, S. M., LaPointe, N. M. A., Kramer, J. M., & Califf, R. M. (2003). What clinicians should know about the QT interval. *JAMA, 289*(16), 2120–2127.

Allison, P. S. (1998). Cardiac anatomy and physiology. In S. Paul & J. D. Hebra (Eds.), *The nurse's guide to cardiac rhythm interpretation. Implications for patient care* (pp. 3–13). Philadelphia: Saunders.

Alpert, J. S., Thygesen, K., Antman, E., & Bassand, J. P. (2000). Myocardial infarction redefined: A consensus document of the Joint European Society of Cardiology/American College of Cardiology Committee for the redefinition of myocardial infarction. *Journal of American College of Cardiology, 36*(3), 959–969.

American Heart Association. (2007a). *AV junctional rhythm disturbances.* Retrieved June 15, 2008, from http://www.americanheart.org/presenter.jhtml?identifier=746

American Heart Association. (2007b). *Cardiac conduction system.* Retrieved June 4, 2008, from http://www.americanheart.org/presenter.jhtml?identifier=68

American Heart Association. (2007c). *Electrocardiogram (EKG or ECG)*. Retrieved March 8, 2008, from http://www.americanheart.org/presenter.jhtml?identifier=3005172

American Heart Association. (2007d). *Sinus disturbances*. Retrieved June 14, 2008, from http://www.americanheart.org/presenter.jhtml?identifier=55

American Heart Association. (2007e). *Ventricular tachycardia*. Retrieved June 4, 2008, from http://www.americanheart.org/presenter.jhtml?identifier=64

American Heart Association Guidelines for Cardiopulmonary Resuscitation and Emergency Cardiovascular Care. (2005). *Circulation, 112*(Suppl. 24), IV, 1–89. Baltimore: Lippincott Williams & Wilkins.

American Heart Association Handbook of Emergency Cardiovascular Care for Healthcare Providers. (2008). Dallas, TX: American Heart Association.

Andreasen, J. B., Johnsen, S. P., & Ravn, H. B. (2008). Junctional ectopic tachycardia after surgery for congenital heart disease in children. *Intensive Care Medicine, 34*(5), 895–902. Retrieved August 3, 2008, from http://www.ncbi.nlm.nih.gov/pubmed/18196218?dopt=AbstractPlus

Ariyarajah, V., Mercado, K., Apiyasawat, S., Puri, P., & Spodick, D. H. (2005). Correlation of left atrial size with p-wave duration in interatrial block. *Chest, 128*(4), 2615–2618. Retrieved March 20, 2008, from ProQuest Nursing & Allied Health Source.

Arnsdorf, M. F. (n.d.). *Left median (middle or septal fascicular block)*. Retrieved March 14, 2008, from http://patients.uptodate.com/topic.asp?file=ecgs/7775

Bargout, R., & Lucas, B. P. (2002). The clinical picture: A homeless 63 year old man with an abnormal electrocardiogram. *Cleveland Clinic Journal of Medicine, 69*(1), 62–64. Retrieved July 14, 2008, from http://www.ccjm.org/pdffiles/Bargout1-02.pdf

Bhatia, V., & Kaul, U. (2007). Common errors in ECG diagnosis of coronary artery disease. *Journal of the Association of Physicians of India, 55*(Suppl.), 7–9. Retrieved June 2, 2008, from http://www.japi.org/april2007/suppliment/Suppliment_07-09.pdg

Bjerregaard, P., & Collier, J. (2004–2007). Short QT syndrome. Retrieved December 10, 2008, from http://www.shortqtsyndrome.org/contactinfo.htm

Booker, K. J., Holm, K., Drew, B. J., Lanuza, D. M., Hicks, F. D., Carrigan, T., et al. (2003). Frequency and outcomes of transient myocardial ischemia in critically ill adults admitted for noncardiac conditions. *American Journal of Critical Care, 12*(6), 508–516.

Bresnahan, S., & Eastwood, J. (2007). Confounding T-wave inversion. *American Journal of Critical Care, 16*(2), 137–140.

Brugada syndrome. (n.d.). *Diagnosis*. Retrieved May 28, 2008, from http://www.brugada.org/about/disease-diagnosis.html

Cardiology: Discovery of the electrical system of the heart presented in an historical perspective. (2006). *Obesity, Fitness, & Wellness,* 605. Retrieved March 12, 2008, from ProQuest Nursing & Allied Health Source.

Carter, T., & Ellis, K. (2005). Right ventricular infarction. *Critical Care Nurse, 25*(2), 52–62.

Casey, P. E., Morrissey, A., & Nolan, E. M. (1996). Ischemic heart disease. In M. R. Kinney, S. B. Dunbar, J. B. Brooks-Brunn, N. Molter, & J. M. Vitello-Cicciu (Eds.), *AACN's clinical reference for critical care nursing* (4th ed., pp. 319–381). St. Louis, MO: Mosby.

Castellanos, A., Pastor, J. A., Zambrano, J. P., & Myerburg, R. J. (2002). Left bundle-branch block with technical right axis deviation. *Circulation, 106*, 2288. Retrieved May 14, 2008, from http://www.circ.ahajournals.org/cgi/content/full/106/17/2288

Clark, R. K. (2005). *Anatomy and physiology. Understanding the human body.* Sudbury, MA: Jones and Bartlett.

Conover, M. B. (2003). *Understanding electrocardiography* (8th ed.). St. Louis, MO: Mosby.

*Critical care nursing made incredibly easy.* (2004). Ambler, PA: Lippincott Williams & Wilkins.

Devon, H. A., Ryan, C. J., Ochs, A. L., & Shapiro, M. (2008). Symptoms across the continuum of acute coronary syndromes: Differences between women and men. *American Journal of Critical Care, 17*(1), 14–25.

Diepenbrock, N. H. (2004). *Quick reference to critical care* (2nd ed.). Philadelphia: Lippincott Williams & Wilkins.

Drew, B. J. (2002). Celebrating the 100th birthday of the electrocardiogram: Lessons learned from research in cardiac monitoring. *American Journal of Critical Care, 11*(4), 378–386.

Drew, B. J., & Krucoff, M. W. (1999). Multilead ST-segment monitoring in patients with acute coronary syndromes: A consensus statement for healthcare professionals. *American Journal of Critical Care, 8*(6), 372–376.

Drew, B. J., Pelter, M. M., Adams, M. G., & Wung, S. (1998). 12-lead ST-segment monitoring vs. single-lead maximum ST-segment monitoring for detecting ongoing ischemia in patients with unstable coronary syndromes. *American Journal of Critical Care, 7*(5), 355–363.

Dubin, D. (1996). *Rapid interpretation of EKG's* (5th ed.). Tampa, FL: COVER.

Dubin, D. (2000). *Rapid interpretation of EKG's* (6th ed.). Tampa, FL: COVER.

Eagan, J. S. (1996). Life-threatening dysrhythmias. In M. R. Kinney, S. B. Dunbar, J. B. Brooks-Brunn, N. Molter, & J. M. Vitello-Cicciu (Eds.), *AACN's clinical reference for critical care nursing* (4th ed., pp. 461–488). St. Louis, MO: Mosby.

Edhouse, J., Brady, W. J., & Morris, F. (2002). Acute myocardial infarction: Part 11. *British Medical Journal, 324*(7343), 963–966. Retrieved June 3, 2008, from http://www.pubmedcentral.nih.gov/articlerender.fcgi?artid=1122906

Eskola, M. J., Nikus, K. C., Voipio-Pulkki, L., Huhtala, H., Parviainen, T., Lund, J., et al. (2005). Comparative accuracy of manual versus computerized electrocardiographic measurement of J-, ST- and T-wave deviations in patients with acute coronary syndrome. *American Journal of Cardiology, 96*(11), 1584–1588.

Ezekowitz, M. D. (2007). Maintaining sinus rhythm-making treatment better than the disease. *The New England Journal of Medicine, 357*(10), 1039. Retrieved March 30, 2008, from ProQuest Nursing & Allied Health Source.

Ferguson, T. B., & Cox, J. L. (1995). Surgical treatment of arrhythmias. In J. A. Kruse, M. P. Fink, & R. W. Carlson (Eds.), *Saunders manual of critical care* (pp. 1476–1494). Philadelphia: Saunders.

Flanders, S. A. (2007). ST-segment monitoring: Putting standards into practice. *AACN Advanced Critical Care, 18*(3), 275–284.

Ganz, L. I. (2003). Approach to the patient with asymptomatic electrocardiographic abnormalities. In E. Braunwald & L. Goldman (Eds.), *Primary cardiology* (2nd ed., pp. 169–192). Philadelphia: Saunders.

Garcia, T. B., & Holtz, N. E. (2001). *12-lead ECG. The art of interpretation.* Sudbury, MA: Jones and Bartlett.

Geiter, H. B. (2003). Understanding bundle-branch blocks. *Nursing, 33*(4), 32cc1–32cc5. Retrieved March 31, 2008, from ProQuest Nursing & Allied Health Source.

Gersh, B. J. (Ed.). (2000). *Mayo Clinic heart book.* New York: William Morrow.

Gilbert, M., & Wagner, G. S. (2008a). Re-entrant junctional tachyarrhythmias. In G. S. Wagner (Ed.), *Marriott's practical electrocardiography* (11th ed., pp. 328–345). Philadelphia: Lippincott Williams & Wilkins.

Gilbert, M., & Wagner, G. S. (2008b). Re-entrant ventricular tachyarrhythmias. In G. S. Wagner (Ed.), *Marriott's practical electrocardiography* (11th ed., pp. 348–369). Philadelphia: Lippincott Williams & Wilkins.

Goyle, K. K., & Walling, A. D. (2002). Diagnosing pericarditis. *American Family Physician, 66*(9), 1695–1702. Retrieved June 2, 2008, from http://www.aafp.org/afp/20021101/1695.html

Haberl, R. (2002–2005). *ECG pocket: Clinical reference guide.* Hermosa Beach, CA: Börm Bruckmeier Publishing.

Haissaguerre, M., Derval, N., Sacher, F., Jesel, L., Deisenhofer, I., Roy, L., et al. (2008). Sudden cardiac arrest associated with early repolarization [Abstract], *The New England Journal of Medicine, 19*(358), 2016–2023. Retrieved December 7, 2008, from http://content.nejm.org/cgi/content/abstract/358/19/2016

Hayes, D. L. (1993). Indications for permanent pacing. In S. Furman, D. L. Hayes, & D. R. Holmes (Eds.), *A practice of cardiac pacing* (3rd ed., pp. 1–28). Mount Kisco, NY: Futura Publishing.

Hayes, D. L., & Holmes, D. R. (1993). Temporary cardiac pacing. In S. Furman, D. L. Hayes, & D. R. Holmes (Eds.), *A practice of cardiac pacing* (3rd ed., pp. 231–260). Mount Kisco, NY: Futura Publishing.

Haywood, L. J. (2005). Left bundle branch block in acute myocardial infarction [Editorial Comment]. *Journal of the American College of Cardiology, 46,* 39–41. Retrieved November 30, 2008, from http://content.onlinejacc.org/cgi/content/full/46/1/39

Hebbar, A. K., & Hueston, W. J. (2002). Management of common arrhythmias: Part II. Ventricular arrhythmias and arrhythmias in special populations. *American Family Physician, 65*(12), 2491–2496. Retrieved March 31, 2008, from ProQuest Nursing & Allied Health Source.

Hebra, J. D. (1998). Basic concepts in rhythm interpretation. In S. Paul & J. D. Hebra (Eds.), *The nurse's guide to cardiac rhythm interpretation* (pp. 22–39). Philadelphia: Saunders.

Heidbuchel, H., & Jackman, W. M. (2004). Characterization of subforms of AV nodal reentrant tachycardia. *Europace, 6*(4), 316–329. Retrieved July 22, 2008, from http://europace.oxfordjournals.org/cgi/content/full/6/4/316

Heiseman, D. L. (2007). *Cardiac rhythm interpretation.* Retrieved April 4, 2008, from http://www.free-ed.net/sweethaven/MedTech/ CardiacRhythm/571.asp?iNum0102

Homoud, M. K. (2008). *Introduction to electrocardiography.* Retrieved April 5, 2008, from http:// http://ocw.tufts.edu/data/50/636805.pdf

Horenstein, M. S. (2008). *Supraventricular tachycardia, junctional ectopic tachycardia.* Retrieved July 25, 2008, from http://www.emedicine.com/ped/topic2536.htm

Jacobson, C. (2007). Narrow QRS complex tachycardias. *AACN Advanced Critical Care, 18*(3), 264–274. Retrieved April 4, 2008, from Ovid database.

Jahrsdoerfer, M., Guiliano, K., & Stephens, D. (2005). Clinical usefulness of the EASI 12-lead continuous electrocardiographic monitoring system. *Critical Care Nurse, 25*(5), 28–37. Retrieved June 2, 2008, from http://ccn.aacnjournals.org/cgi/reprint/25/5/28.pdf

Katritis, D. G., & Camm, A. J. (2006). Classification and differential diagnosis of atrioventricular nodal re-entrant tachycardia. *Europace, 8*(1), 29–36. Retrieved July 22, 2008, from http://europace.oxfordjournals.org/cgi/content/full/8/1/29

Keller, K. B. (2008). Torsade. *Critical Care Nurse, 17*(1), 77–81.

Kern, L. S., McRae, M. E., & Funk, M. (2007). ECG monitoring after cardiac surgery: Postoperative atrial fibrillation and the atrial electrocardiogram. *AACN Advanced Critical Care, 18*(3), 294–307. Retrieved April 14, 2008, from Ovid database.

Klabunde, R. E. (1999–2007). *Electrocardiogram.* Retrieved April 3, 2008, from http://www.cvphysiology.com/CAD/CAD012.htm

Kligfield, P., Gettes, L. S., Bailey, J. J., Childers, R., Deal, B. J., Hancock, W., et al. (2007a). Recommendations for the standardization and interpretation of the electrocardiogram. Part1: The electrocardiogram and its technology. A scientific statement from the American Heart Association Electrocardiography and Arrhythmias committee, Council on Clinical Cardiology, the American College of Cardiology Foundation, and the Heart Rhythm Society. *Circulation, 115,* 1306–1324. Retrieved May 30, 2008, from http://www.circ.ahajournals.org/cgi/content/abstract/115/10/1306

Kramer, M. J., Ide, B., & Drew, B. J. (1999). What is the most common arrhythmia following cardiac revascularization? *Progress in Cardiovascular Nursing, 14*(4), 159–161. Retrieved April 9, 2008, from ProQuest Nursing & Allied Health Source.

Kupersmith, J. (1993). Long QT syndrome. In I. Singer & J. Kupersmith (Eds.), *Clinical manual of electrophysiology* (pp. 143–168). Baltimore: Williams & Wilkins.

Langfitt, D. E. (1984). *Critical care certification preparation & review.* Bowie, MD: Robert J. Brady.

Levin, T. (2008). *Right ventricular myocardial infarction.* Retrieved May 18, 2008, from http://www.uptodate.com/patients/content/topic.do? topickey=chd/2454

Lip, G. Y. H., & Tse, H. (2007). Management of atrial fibrillation. *The Lancet, 370*(9587), 604–618. Retrieved March 22, 2008, from ProQuest Nursing & Allied Health Source.

Lisbon, A., & Fink, M. P. (2003). Post-cardiac surgery management. In J. A. Kruse, M. P. Fink, & R. W. Carlson (Eds.), *Saunders manual of critical care* (pp. 500–503). Philadelphia: Saunders.

Livingston, J. C., Mabie, B. C., & Ramanathan, J. (2000). Crack cocaine, myocardial infarction, and troponin I levels at the time of cesarean delivery. *Anesthesia & Analgesia, 91*, 913–915. Retrieved July 16, 2008, from http://www.anesthesia-analgesia.org/cgi/content/full/91/4/913

Lloyd, M. A., & Hayes, D. L. (2000). Pacemakers. In J. G. Murphy (Ed.), *Mayo Clinic cardiology review* (2nd ed., pp. 669–684). Philadelphia: Lippincott Williams & Wilkins.

Marinella, M. A. (1998). Electrocardiographic manifestations and differential diagnosis of acute pericarditis. *American Family Physician, 57*(4), 703. Retrieved July 13, 2008, from http://www.aafp.org/afp/980215ap/marinell.html

Mascitelli, L., & Pezzetta, F. (2006). Case report: Differentiating artifact from true ventricular tachycardia [Letter to the editor]. *American Family Physician, 74*(6), 921. Retrieved May 18, 2008, from ProQuest Nursing & Allied Health Source.

Mayo Clinic. (2005). Researchers discover genetic glitch in the heart's electrical system. *Biotech Week*, 632. Retrieved March 14, 2008, from ProQuest Nursing & Allied Health Source.

McAvoy, J. (2004). Case studies of ST segment elevation before and after percutaneous coronary intervention in patients with acute MI. *Critical Care Nurse, 24*(6), 32–39. Retrieved April 4, 2008, from http://cccn.aacnjournals.org/cgi/content/full/24/6/32

McCord, J., & Borzak, S. (1998). Multifocal atrial tachycardia [Abstract]. *Chest, 113*(1), 203–209. Retrieved August 1, 2008, from http://www.ncbi.nlm.nih.gov/pubmed/9440591

Mishell, J. M., & Goldschlager, N. (2003). Recognition and management of patients with bradyarrhythmias. In E. Braunwald & L. Goldman (Eds.), *Primary cardiology* (2nd ed., pp. 529–551). Philadelphia: Saunders.

Murphy, J. G. (2000a). Applied anatomy of the heart and the great vessels. In J. G. Murphy (Ed.), *Mayo Clinic cardiology review* (2nd ed., pp. 927–960). Philadelphia: Lippincott Williams & Wilkins.

Murphy, J. G. (2000b). Coronary angioplasty in myocardial infarction. In J. G. Murphy (Ed.), *Mayo Clinic cardiology review* (2nd ed., pp. 193–208). Philadelphia: Lippincott Williams & Wilkins.

Naccarelli, G. V., Willerson, J. T., & Blomqvist, C. G. (1995). Recognition and physiologic treatment of cardiac arrhythmias and conduction disturbances. In J. T. Willerson & J. N. Cohn (Eds.), *Cardiovascular medicine* (pp. 1282–1295). New York: Churchill Livingston.

Nair, R., & Glancy, D. L. (2002). ECG discrimination between right and left circumflex coronary arterial occlusion in patients with acute inferior myocardial infarction. *Chest, 122*(1), 134–139. Retrieved March 23, 2008, from ProQuest Nursing & Allied Health Source.

National Guideline Clearinghouse. (1998–2008). *Diagnosis and treatment of chest pain and acute coronary syndrome (ACS)*. Retrieved June 3, 2008, from http://www.guideline.gov/summary/summary.aspx?doc-id=10227

National Heart Lung and Blood Institute. (n.d.). *How are arrhythmias diagnosed?* Retrieved December 11, 2008, from http://www.nhlbi.nih.gov/health/dci/Diseases/arr/arr_diagnosis.html

Nattel, S., Burstein, B., & Dobrev, D. (2008). Atrial remodeling and atrial fibrillation. *Circulation: Arrhythmia and Electrophysiology, 1*(1), 62–73. Retrieved April 25, 2008, from http://circep.ahajournals.org/cgi/content/full/1/1/62

Neill, J., Shannon, H. J., Morton, A., Muir, A. R., Harbinson, M., & Adgey, J. A. (2007). ST segment elevation in lead aVR during exercise testing is associated with LAD stenosis. *European Journal of Nuclear Medicine and Molecular Imaging, 34*(3), 338–345. Retrieved April 30, 2008, from ProQuest Nursing & Allied Health Source.

Nichols, R. L. (2001). *Preventing surgical site infections: A surgeon's perspective.* Retrieved July 19, 2008, from http://www.cdc.gov/ncidod/eid/vol7no2/nichols.htm

Nishimura, R. A., & Kidd, K. R. (2003). Recognition and management of patients with pericardial disease. In E. Braunwald & L. Goldman (Eds.), *Primary cardiology* (2nd ed., pp. 625–642). Philadelphia: Saunders.

Packer, D. L. (2000). Normal and abnormal cardiac electrophysiology. In J. G. Murphy (Ed.), *Mayo Clinic cardiology review* (2nd ed., pp. 699–712). Philadelphia: Lippincott Williams & Wilkins.

Paul, S. (1998). Sinus rhythms. In S. Paul & J. D. Hebra (Eds.), *The nurse's guide to cardiac rhythm interpretation* (pp. 59–79). Philadelphia: Saunders.

Pelter, M. M., Adams, M. G., & Drew, B. J. D. (2002). Association of transient myocardial ischemia with adverse in-hospital outcomes for angina patients treated in a telemetry unit or a coronary care unit. *American Journal of Critical Care, 11*(4), 318–325. Retrieved May 20, 2008, from http://ajcc.aacnjournals.org/cgi/content/full/11/4/318

Pelter, M. M., & Carey, M. G. (2007). P wave alterations. *American Journal of Critical Care, 16*(2), 187–188.

Poglagen, G., Fister, M., Radorancevic, B., & Vrtovec, B. (2006). Short QT interval and atrial fibrillation without structural heart disease [Letter to the Editor]. *Journal of American College of Cardiology, 47,* 1905–1907. Retrieved December 10, 2008, from http://content.onlinejacc.org/cgi/reprint/47/9/1905.pdf

Poliac, L. C., Barron, M. E., & Maron, B. J. (2006). Hypertrophic cardiomyopathy. *Anesthesiology, 104*(1), 183–192.

Porter, W. (2007). *Pocket guide to emergency and critical care.* Sudbury, MA: Jones and Bartlett.

Pugh, M. B. (2000). *Stedman's medical dictionary* (27th ed.). Baltimore: Lippincott Williams & Wilkins.

Rauen, C. A., Chulay, M., Bridges, E., Vollman, K. M., & Arbour, R. (2008). Seven evidence-based practice habits: Putting some sacred cows out to pasture. *Critical Care Nurse, 28*(2), 98–123.

Reinig, M. G., & Engel, T. R. (2007). *The shortage of short QTs. Chest.* Retrieved December 10, 2008, from http://www.chestjournal.org/cgi/reprint/chest.06-2133v1

Riezebos, R. K., Man, K., Patterson, M. S., & Ruiter, G. S. (2007). Case report: A bridge to brugada. *Europace, 9,* 398–400. Retrieved June 3, 2008, from http://europace.oxfordjounals.org/cgi/reprint/9/6/398.pdf

Sakata, K., Shimizu, M., Ino, H., Yamaguchi, M., Terai, H., Hayashi, K., et al. (2003). QT dispersion and left ventricular morphology in patients with hypertrophic cardiomyopathy. *Heart, 89*(8), 882–886. Retrieved March 31, 2008, from ProQuest Nursing & Allied Health Source.

Salles, G., Cardoso, C., Noqueira, A. R., Bloch, K., & Muxfeldt, E. (2006). Importance of the electrocardiographic strain pattern in patients with resistant hypertension. *Hypertension, 48*, 437–442. Retrieved July 13, 2008, from http://hyper.ahajournals.org/cgi/content/full/48/3/437

Sangrigoli, R., & Hsia, H. H. (2002). Cardiac arrhythmias. In G. J. Criner & G. E. D'Alonzo (Eds.), *Critical care study guide text and review* (pp. 241–266). New York: Springer-Verlag.

Scheinman, M. M., & Kaushik, V. (2003). Recognition and management of patients with tachyarrhythmias. In E. Braunwald & L. Goldman (Eds.), *Primary cardiology* (2nd ed., pp. 503–528). Philadelphia: Saunders.

Sgarbossa, E. B., Pinski, S. L., Barbagelata, A., Underwood, D. A., Gates, K. B., Topol, E. J., et al. (1996a). Electrocardiographic diagnosis of evolving acute myocardial infarction in the presence of a left bundle branch block. *New England Journal of Medicine, 334*(8), 481–487. Retrieved July 19, 2008, from http://content.nejm.org/cgi/content/full/334/8/481

Sgarbossa, E. B., Pinski, S. L., Barbagelata, A., Underwood, D. A., Gates, K. B., Topol, E. J., et al. (1996b). Electrocardiographic diagnosis of evolving acute myocardial infarction in the presence of a left bundle branch block [Correction]. *New England Journal of Medicine, 334*(14), 931. Retrieved July 19, 2008, from http://content.nejm.org/cgi/content/full/334/14/931

Shaughnessy, K. (2007). Massive pulmonary embolism. *Critical Care Nurse, 27*(1), 39–50.

Smith, R. N. (1996). Concepts of monitoring and surveillance. In M. R. Kinney, S. B. Dunbar, J. B. Brooks-Brunn, N. Molter, & J. M. Vitello-Cicciu (Eds.), *AACN's clinical reference for critical care nursing* (4th ed., pp. 3–37). St. Louis, MO: Mosby.

Soghoian, S., Doty, C. I., Maffei, F. A., & Connolly, H. (2006). *Toxicity, tricyclic antidepressant*. Retrieved July 16, 2008, from http://www.emedicine.com/ped/topic2714.htm

Solomon, S. D. (2003). Principles of echocardiography. In E. Braunwald & L. Goldman (Eds.), *Primary cardiology* (2nd ed., pp. 63–80). Philadelphia: Saunders.

Sommargren, C. E., & Drew, B. J. (2007). Preventing torsade de pointes by careful cardiac monitoring in hospital settings. *AACN Advanced Critical Care, 18*(3), 285–293.

Sovari, A. A., Prasun, M. A., & Kocheril, A. G. (2007). ST segment elevation on electrocardiogram. The electrocardiographic pattern of Brugada syndrome. *Medscape General Medicine, 9*(3), 59. Retrieved June 2, 2008, from http://www.pubmedcentral.nih.gov/articlerender.fcgi?artid=2100131

Stephens-Lesser, D. (2007). *Cardiac surgery manual for nurses. Orientation, policy, and procedures*. Sudbury, MA: Jones and Bartlett.

Stewart, S. L., & Vitello-Cicciu, J. M. (1996). Cardiovascular clinical physiology. In M. R. Kinney, S. B. Dunbar, J. B. Brooks-Brunn, N. Molter, & J. M. Vitello-Cicciu (Eds.), *AACN's clinical reference for critical care nursing* (4th ed., pp. 249–276). St. Louis, MO: Mosby.

Strasburger, J. F., Cuneo, B. F., Michon, M. M., Gotteiner, N. L., Deal, B. J., McGregor, S. N., et al. (2004). Amiodarone therapy for drug-refractory fetal tachycardia. *Circulation, 109*, 375–379. Retrieved July 25, 2008, from http://circ.ahajournals.org/cgi/reprint/109/3/375.pdf

Taggart, N. W., Haglund, C. M., Tester, D. J., & Ackerman, M. J. (2007). Diagnostic miscues in congenital long-QT syndrome. *Circulation, 115*, 2613–2620. Retrieved March 31, 2008, from ProQuest Nursing & Allied Health Source.

Tan, H. L., & Meregalli, P. G. (2007). Lethal ECG changes hidden by therapeutic hypothermia. *The Lancet, 369*(9555), 78. Retrieved May 12, 2008, from ProQuest Nursing & Allied Health Source.

The Society for Cardiological Science & Technology. (2006). *Clinical guidelines by consensus. Recording a standard 12-lead electrocardiogram. An approved methodology.* Retrieved May 25, 2008, from http://www.scst.org.uk/docs/Consensus_guideline_for_recording_a_12_lead_ECG_2006.pdf

Thygesen, K., Alpert, J. S., & White, H. D. (2007). Universal definition of myocardial infarction. *Journal of the American College of Cardiology, 50*, 2173–2195. Retrieved May 27, 2008, from http://content.onlinejacc.org/cgi/content/full/j.jacc.2007.09.011

Twedell, D. (2005). An overview of congenital long QT syndrome. *The Journal of Continuing Education in Nursing, 36*(1), 14–15. Retrieved March 31, 2008, from ProQuest Nursing & Allied Health Source.

U.S. National Library of Medicine. (2008). *Brugada syndrome*. Retrieved June 10, 2008, from http://ghr.nlm.nih.gov/condition=brugadasyndrome

U.S. National Library of Medicine. (2008). *Short QT syndrome*. Retrieved December 10, 2008, from http://ghr.nlm.nih.gov/condition=shortqtsyndrome

Vacek, J. L. (2002). Classic Q wave myocardial infarction; aggressive, early intervention has dramatic results. *Postgraduate Medicine, 112*(1), 71. Retrieved March 23, 2008, from ProQuest Nursing & Allied Health Source.

Wagner, G. S. (2008). Re-entrant atrial tachyarrhythmias: The atrial flutter/fibrillation spectrum. In G. S. Wagner (Ed.), *Marriott's practical electrocardiography* (11th ed., pp. 302–326). Philadelphia: Lippincott Williams & Wilkins.

Wagner, G. S., & Lim, T. H. (2008a). Interpretation of the normal electrocardiogram. In G. S. Wagner (Ed.), *Marriott's practical electrocardiography* (11th ed., pp. 44–70). Philadelphia: Lippincott Williams & Wilkins.

Wagner, G. S., & Lim, T. H. (2008b). Chamber enlargement. In G. S. Wagner (Ed.), *Marriott's practical electrocardiography* (11th ed., pp. 71–96). Philadelphia: Lippincott Williams & Wilkins.

Wagner, G. S., Selvester, R. H., White, R. D., & Wagner, N. B. (1995). Twelve-lead ECG and extent of myocardium at risk of acute infarction. In R. M. Califf, D. B. Mark, & G. S. Wagner (Eds.), *Acute coronary care* (2nd ed., pp. 229–245). St. Louis, MO: Mosby.

Wagner, G. S., & Wang, T. Y. (2008a). Accelerated automaticity. In G. S. Wagner (Ed.), *Marriott's practical electrocardiography* (11th ed., pp. 288–326). Philadelphia: Lippincott Williams & Wilkins.

Wagner, G. S., & Wang, T. Y. (2008b). Miscellaneous conditions. In G. S. Wagner (Ed.), *Marriott's practical electrocardiography* (11th ed., pp. 210–237). Philadelphia: Lippincott Williams & Wilkins.

Walling, A. D. (2006). Q waves predict mortality in myocardial infarction. *American Family Physician, 74*(9), 1609–1610. Retrieved May 18, 2008, from ProQuest Nursing & Allied Health Source.

Win-Kuang, S. (2000). Cardiac cellular electrophysiology. In J. G. Murphy (Ed.), *Mayo Clinic cardiology review* (2nd ed., pp. 597–620). Philadelphia: Lippincott Williams & Wilkins.

Wong, C., French, J. K., Aylward, P. E. G., Stewart, R. A. H., Wanzhen, G., Armstrong, P. W., et al. (2005). Patients with prolonged ischemic chest pain and presumed-new left bundle branch block have heterogeneous outcomes depending on the presence of ST-segment changes. *Journal of the American College of Cardiology, 46,* 29–31. Retrieved November 30, 2008, from http://content.onlinejacc.org/cgi/content/full/46/1/29#TBL3

Zaccheo, M. M., & Bucher, D. H. (2008). Propofol infusion syndrome. A rare complication with potentially fatal results. *Critical Care Nurse, 28*(3), 18–25.

Zeigler, V. L., & Gillette, P. C. (2001). *Practical management of pediatric cardiac arrhythmias.* Blackwell. Retrieved August 3, 2008, from http://books.google.com/books?hl=en&lr=&id=1YiI9F7R7dEC&oi=fnd&pg=PP7&dq=practical+management+of+pediatric+arrhythmias+and+google+books&ots=Lp2Utd_i0V&sig=3oHIz4T4-liROvXlV67TT4JdjKs#PPA81,M

# Index